Viviannie Amélia de Aquino Cardoso

PHARMACEUTICAL MANAGEMENT IN ONCOLOGY AND HEMATOLOGY

Viviannie Amélia de Aquino Cardoso

PHARMACEUTICAL MANAGEMENT IN ONCOLOGY AND HEMATOLOGY

A COLLECTION OF CHEMOTHERAPY PROTOCOLS

ScienciaScripts

Imprint
Any brand names and product names mentioned in this book are subject to trademark, brand or patent protection and are trademarks or registered trademarks of their respective holders. The use of brand names, product names, common names, trade names, product descriptions etc. even without a particular marking in this work is in no way to be construed to mean that such names may be regarded as unrestricted in respect of trademark and brand protection legislation and could thus be used by anyone.

Cover image: www.ingimage.com

This book is a translation from the original published under ISBN 978-620-5-50617-2.

Publisher:
Sciencia Scripts
is a trademark of
Dodo Books Indian Ocean Ltd. and OmniScriptum S.R.L publishing group

120 High Road, East Finchley, London, N2 9ED, United Kingdom
Str. Armeneasca 28/1, office 1, Chisinau MD-2012, Republic of Moldova, Europe
Printed at: see last page
ISBN: 978-620-6-18899-5

I thank God for the opportunity to live, the teachers who have passed through my educational path, for the diffusing source of knowledge, and, last but not least, my parents, Antônio Francisco Cardoso and Vilma Conceição de Aquino, and my brothers Germano Cardoso Neto and Hugo Antônio de Aquino Cardoso for the strength they have always given me.

My sincere thanks.

"Every effect has a cause. Every intelligent effect has an intelligent cause. The power of the intelligent cause is in the ratio of the greatness of the effect."

Allan Kardec

"Wisdom is a solid and unique construction, in which each part has its place and makes its mark."

Michel Eyquem de Montaigne

PRESENTATION

This Pharmaceutical Manuscript is a compilation of standardized Hormonotherapeutic, Chemotherapeutic and Immunotherapeutic Drugs with the role of providing safe and updated information for the use of Hormonotherapeutic, Chemotherapeutic and Immunotherapeutic Drugs and to facilitate the availability of this information for everyone's access. It will include 55 active ingredients in alphabetical order with information on the commercial name, pharmaceutical form, usual dose *(the usual dose is only a form of guidance for the transdisciplinary team, leaving it to the discretion of the physician to decide the appropriate dose for the patient)*, guidelines for preparation, stability, administration, and dosage adjustment, and for each drug a study will be presented, in which the pharmacological aspects, effectiveness, therapeutic safety, pharmacokinetics, pharmacotechnics, epidemiology, and pharmacoeconomics are referenced.

INTRODUCTION

According to the National Cancer Institute (INCA), Cancer is the name given to a group of more than 100 diseases that have in common the disordered (malignant) growth of cells that invade tissues and organs, and can spread (metastasize) to other regions of the body.

When these cells divide rapidly, they tend to be very aggressive and uncontrollable, leading to the formation of tumors (accumulation of cancerous cells) or malignant neoplasms. On the other hand, a benign tumor simply means a localized mass of cells that multiply slowly and resemble their original tissue, and are rarely life-threatening.

There are different types of cancer which correspond to the various types of cells in the body. Characteristics that differentiate the various types of cancer from one another are the speed at which the cells multiply and the ability to invade neighboring or distant tissues and organs (metastasis).

Cancer has several causes, which can be both external and internal to the organism, and both are interrelated. External causes are related to the environment and to the habits or customs of a social and cultural environment. Internal causes are, most of the time, genetically predetermined, and are linked to the organism's capacity to defend itself from external aggressions. These causal factors can interact in various ways, increasing the probability of malignant transformations in normal cells.

The cells that make up animals are made up of three parts: the cell membrane, which is the outermost part; the cytoplasm (the body of the cell); and the nucleus, which contains the chromosomes, which, in turn, are composed of genes. Genes are files that store and provide instructions for the organization of the structures, shapes and activities of cells in the organism. All genetic information is inscribed in the genes in a "chemical memory" - deoxyribonucleic acid (DNA). It is through DNA that the chromosomes pass the information for the functioning of the cell. A normal cell can undergo changes in the DNA of genes.

This is what we call genetic mutation. Cells whose genetic material has been altered are given the wrong instructions for their activities. The changes can occur in special genes, called protooncogenes, which are initially inactive in normal cells. When activated, the protooncogenes become oncogenes, which are responsible for the malignancy (cancerization) of normal cells. These different cells are called cancer cells.

It is known that changes are always part of our lives, some are planned, others not, some are desired, others not; any change brings the need to deal with the new, with the unknown. For those who are sick, needing long treatments, with integral and differentiated assistance and with several special cares, changes in their life routine and also in that of their family are required. There are no rules or fixed ways to deal with new situations; each person and family has its own way of being, facing and dealing with problems.

It is natural at the beginning of a chemotherapy treatment to have different reactions, feelings, and questions. At this beginning, discomfort and strangeness may occur, both due to physical discomfort and to the abrupt change of environment. Chemotherapy is a type of treatment used in individuals with neoplasms, which consists of the use of drugs that act by destroying the sick cells.

Often, two or more drugs are used in combination. The rationale behind combination chemotherapy is to use drugs that act on different parts of the metabolic processes of the cell, thus increasing the chance of destroying a greater number of diseased cells. In addition, it allows the doses of each drug to be smaller, reducing toxicity and side effects.

Chemotherapy can be by route:

Oral - pills that you can take home;
Intravenous - in the vein; by needles or catheters;
Intramuscular - injections into the muscle;
Subcutaneous - injections under the skin;
Intrathecal - injections into the spinal canal, via lumbar puncture.

Chemotherapy drugs can cause some side effects, which depend on the type of drug used and the phase of treatment. The most common are nausea, vomiting, and a decrease in the number of blood cells, which can lead to anemia due to a decrease in the number of red blood cells, bleeding due to a decrease in the number of platelets, and infections due to a decrease in the number of white blood cells.

CONTENT

MEDICINES

FOLINIC ACID

Trade Name/Presentation: Calcium Folinate: Ampoule bottle with 300mg/30mL or 50mg lyophilized powder.

Fauldleuco: Ampoule vial in dosage 50 mg/5 mL

Prevax: 15mg/tablet

Therapeutic Category: Antidote

Indication: Antidote to folic acid antagonists (e.g. methotrexate >100mg/m2); treatment of megaloblastic anemias when folate is deficient, as in infancy, pregnancy, or when folate therapy is not possible; in combination with fluorouracil in the treatment of neoplasms.

Usual Dose: Adults and Children: Methotrexate rescue therapy. Rescue therapy should be started as soon as possible, within 24h of MTX administration: 15mg (10mg/m2), IV/IM/VO, every 6h, for 72h, until the serum MTX level is less than 10-8M. If in 24h the serum creatinine increases 50% beyond the baseline value or if the MTX level is greater than 5x10-5M, or if in 48h, the level is greater than 9x10-7M, the leucovorin dose should be adjusted to 100mg/m2, IV, every 3h, until the MTX level is less than 10-8M. Folate deficiency megaloblastic anemia: 1mg/day, IM. Megaloblastic anemia secondary to congenital dihydrofolate reductase deficiency: 3-6mg/day, IM.

Storage: Vials ampoules: 24h RT or under refrigeration. Tablets: TA.

Route of administration/infusion time: IV. Do not exceed 160mg/min.

Use simple equipo.

Reconstitution: Ready for use. Vials of 50 mg lyophilized powder with ABD.

Stability after reconstitution: 24h under refrigeration, only 300 mg presentation, Fauldleuco: 48 Hs under refrigeration.

Dilution: Dilute in 100mL (up to 300mg) and 250mL for doses higher than 300mg.

Stability after dilution: 24h under refrigeration, but it is recommended to use immediately after preparation, since the solution does not contain preservatives.

Recommendations: The tablets can be taken with or without food.

Main Adverse Reactions: Anaphylactoid reactions and urticaria have been reported in the use of folinic acid alone. Concomitant use with 5-FU: Diarrhea, Stomatitis. Leukopenia.

ZOLEDRONIC ACID

Trade Name/Presentation: ZOMETA: Ampoule containing lyophilized powder in dosage of 4 mg and diluent in dosage of 5 mL.

Therapeutic Class: Bone Resorption Inhibitors.

Indication: treatment of tumor-induced hypercalcemia.

Usual Dose: Adults: (albumin-corrected serum calcium $\geq$12.0mg/dL or 3 mmol/L) - 4mg, IV.

Storage: Room temperature.

Route of administration/infusion time: Endovenous under continuous infusion of 15 minutes (strictly).

Use simple equipo.

Reconstitution: Diluent proper.

Stability after reconstitution: Use immediately.

Dilution: Nacl 0.9% or SGI 5%.

Stability after dilution: 24h under refrigeration.

Recommendations: Do not mix the reconstituted solution with calcium-containing solutions, such as Ringer's solution. Renal insufficiency: For patients with creatinine clearance lower than 60ml/min, the dose should range from 3 to 3.5mg of zoledronic acid, diluted in 100mL.

Major Adverse Reactions: Mild and transient. Very common: Hypophosphatemia. Common: anemia, headache, nausea, vomiting, anorexia, fever, flu-like syndrome. Uncommon: Dizziness, paretesias, tremors, skin rash.

MEGESTROL ACETATE

Trade Name/Presentation: Megestat 160mg/tablet.

Therapeutic Category: Antineoplastic, Hormone

Indication: Breast cancer, treatment of anorexia and weight loss related to cancer or AIDS.

Usual Dose: 160 to 320mg, VO, once a day.

Storage: TA

Route of administration/infusion time: Oral

Reconstitution: NA

Stability after reconstitution: NA

Dilution: NA

Stability after dilution: NA

ACTINOMYCIN

Trade Name/Presentation: Cosmegen. Ampoule vial containing 500mcg/flask

Therapeutic Category: Antineoplastic, Antibiotic.

Indication: Wilms' tumor, rhabdomyosarcoma, carcinoma of the testicles and uterus (choriocarcinoma), Kaposi's sarcoma, melanoma, acute non-lymphocytic leukemia, osteosarcoma.

Usual Dose: 10 to 15µg/Kg/day, IV, for 5 days, every 2 to 4 weeks; 100 to 200µg/m2, IV, every 1 to 3 weeks; or 400 to 600µg/m2/day, IV, for 5 days, every 3 to 5 weeks. Children: 400 to 500µg/m2/day, IV, or 10 to 15µg/Kg/day, IV, for 5 days, every 3 to 5 weeks.

Storage: TA

Administration route/infusion time: 3-15 min. Peripheral access: Infuse parallel 250 mL SF.

Use photoresist equipments

Reconstitution: 2 mL ABD

Stability after reconstitution: Immediate use.

Dilution: 20 to 100 mL SF or SG.

Stability after dilution: 24h SR away from light.

Recommendations: Dose Adjustment: Adjustment by liver function: bilirubin > 3mg/Dl - give 50% of the dose. Adjustment by renal function: no data available. Incompatible with preservative-containing diluents. Filgrastim. Infusion filters.

Main Adverse Reactions: Acne. Alopecia (reversible). Myelosuppression. Mucositis. Nausea. Vomiting. Diarrhea Malaise Lethargy.

Recommendations: Great caution in patients with a history of thrombophlebitis. Avoid sun exposure during treatment.

Main Adverse Reactions: Alopecia. Menstrual alterations. Abdominal pain. Dry mouth. Confusion. Constipation. Seizures. Rashes. Skin rash

ANASTROZOLE

Trade Name/Presentation: Arimidex: 1mg/tablet

Therapeutic Class: Antineoplastic, aromatase inhibitor.

Indication: Treatment of early breast cancer in postmenopausal women.

Usual Dose: 1mg, VO, 1 time/day.

Storage: TA

Route of administration/infusion time: NA

Reconstitution: NA

Stability after reconstitution: NA

Dilution: NA

Stability after dilution: NA

Recommendations: The tablet should be administered whole, at the same time every day, with or without food.

Main adverse reactions: ALOPECIA. Anorexia. Weight gain. Headache. Asthenia. Abdominal colic. arthritis constipation depression diarrhea dyspnea pain weakness vaginal bleeding

BEVACIZUMAB

Trade Name/Presentation: Avastin: Single-dose vial of 100 mg (4 mL) or 400 mg (16 mL).

Therapeutic Class: Monoclonal antibody.

Indication: Used in combination with chemotherapy, it is indicated for first-line treatment in patients with carcinoma of the colon and rectum.

Usual Dose: 5 to 10mg/kg every two weeks.

Storage: TA.

Route of administration/Infusion time: Give the first infusion in 90 minutes, the second infusion in 60 minutes, and the next doses in 30 minutes. Administer before chemotherapy.

Simple equipment.

Reconstitution: Ready to use.

Stability after reconstitution: NA.

Dilution: SF 0.9% 100 mL.

Stability after dilution: 24 Hs under refrigeration.

Recommendations: It cannot be administered in bolus. Infusions of Avastin® should not be given into or mixed with dextrose or glucose solutions.

Main adverse reactions: Gastrointestinal perforations. Hemorrhage, including pulmonary hemorrhage / hemoptysis, more common in patients with non-small cell lung cancer. Arterial thromboembolism

BICALUTAMIDE

Trade Name/Presentation: Casodex : 50 mg/tablet

Therapeutic Class: Antineoplastic. Inhibitor of androgenic stimulation

Indication: Advanced (metastatic) prostate cancer and non-metastatic prostate cancer.

Usual Dose: Advanced (metastatic) prostate cancer: - Treatment of advanced prostate cancer in combination with treatment with LHRH analogues or surgical castration : Adults (including the elderly): 1 tablet of 50 mg once daily. Treatment should be started at the same time as treatment with the LHRH analog or surgical castration.

 - Treatment of metastatic prostate cancer in patients in whom surgical or drug castration is not indicated or is not acceptable:

Adults (including the elderly): 3 tablets of 50 mg once a day.

Non-metastatic prostate cancer: Adults (including the elderly): 3 tablets of 50 mg once a day.

Storage: TA

Route of administration/infusion time: Oral.

Reconstitution: NA

Stability after reconstitution: NA

Dilution: NA

Stability after dilution: NA

Recommendations: NA

Main Adverse Reactions: Hot flushes, breast hypersensitivity, nausea, vomiting, diarrhea, itching, and weakness. During treatment with 150 mg a day of CASODEX, the following adverse reactions may occur: breast hypersensitivity, gynecomastia, heat waves, itching, abdominal pain, weakness, depression, nausea, vomiting, hair loss, dry skin, decreased sex drive, and the presence of blood in the urine and changes in the lungs.

BLEOMICIN

Trade Name/Presentation: Bonar: Ampoule containing 15 IU lyophilized powder (15 mg) and 5 mL diluent.

Therapeutic Category: Antineoplastic, Antibiotic

Indication: Palliative. Head and neck squamous cell carcinoma, testicular carcinoma, Hodgkin's and non-Hodgkin's lymphoma and malignant pleural effusion.

Usual Dose: 10 to 20UI/m2, 1-2 times a week.

Storage: Under refrigeration.

Route of administration/infusion time: 10 to 20 IU/m2/day, intra-arterial, in 12- to 24-hour infusion; 60 IU for intrapleural injection. Combination with other agents: IM: 2 to 4 IU/m2; IV: 10 IU/m2, on days 1 and 15 for 10 minutes.

Use simple equipo.

Reconstitution: Diluent proper.

Stability after reconstitution: 24 Hs under refrigeration.

Dilution: 50 - 1000 mL of Nacl 0.9%.

Stability after dilution: 24 Hs under refrigeration.

Recommendations: Before the first and second application, sensitivity testing with 1 to 2 IU of bleomycin, IM or SC, is recommended.

Main Adverse Reactions: Alopecia. Changes in liver and kidney functions. Changes in the nail bed. Prolonged anorexia. Peeling of fingertips. Diarrhea. Dyspnea. erythema rashes Stomatitis and mucositis Nausea and vomiting

CAPECITABINE

Trade Name/Presentation: Xeloda 500mg/tablet

Therapeutic Class: Antineoplastic, Antimetabolite

Indication: locally advanced or metastatic breast cancer, colorectal cancer, and metastatic colorectal cancer.

Usual Dose: 2,500mg/day, VO, 2 times/day (morning and evening), for 2 weeks, followed by 1 week rest. 3-cycle treatment.

Storage: TA

Route of administration/infusion time: Oral.

Reconstitution: NA

Stability after reconstitution: NA

Dilution: NA

Stability after dilution: NA

Recommendations: Tablets should be swallowed with water 30 min after meals. Do not chew and do not macerate.

Main Adverse Reactions: Loss of appetite, diarrhea, vomiting, nausea, mouth sores (stomatitis), abdominal pain, swelling, redness, tingling and numbness of the palms of the hands and soles of the feet, dermatitis, fatigue (tiredness) and lethargy (deep sleep), decreased white blood cells with or without fever, decreased platelets, anemia, altered nerve branches responsible for the sensitivity of hands and feet, taste disturbance, altered sensitivity (numbness or tingling), headache, increased tearing, thrombosis/embolism (clogging of blood vessels by blood clots), high blood pressure, swelling in the legs, sore throat, constipation, stomach upset, hair loss, nail changes, joint pain, muscle pain, pain in the arms and legs, fever, discouragement, weakness, temperature intolerance.

CARBOPLATIN

Trade Name/Presentation: Fauldcarbo: Ampoule vials containing 15 and 45 mL.

Therapeutic Class: Antineoplastic, Alkylating agent.

Indication: Advanced carcinoma of epithelial origin, small cell lung carcinoma, ovarian carcinoma, head and neck cancer, among other indications.

Usual Dose: 300 to 400mg/m2, IV, every 4 weeks; 250mg/m2, if baseline creatinine clearance is between 41 and 59 mL/min; 200mg/m2, if baseline creatinine clearance is between 16 and 40mL/min.

Storage: TA

Route of administration/infusion time: IV from 15 to 120 minutes (usually 60 minutes).

Use photoresist equipments.

Reconstitution: Ready to use.

Stability after reconstitution: 24 h under refrigeration.

Dilution: SS or GS (preferably) in concentration from 0.5mg/mL to 2mg/mL. Usually a concentration of 1mg/mL is used.

Stability after dilution: SF 8 h TA, SG 24 h under refrigeration.

Recommendation: Very high doses of carboplatin (up to five times or more than recommended) have resulted in severe abnormalities in liver and kidney function. Patients previously treated with cisplatin may experience more severe nausea and vomiting. To reduce the incidence and intensity of this adverse event, premedication with antiemetics and prolongation of the carboplatin administration period by continuous infusion or for five consecutive days is recommended.

Main Adverse Reactions: Hypersensitivity and anaphylactic reactions have been reported during therapy with carboplatin and other platinum-containing drugs. These reactions may occur within minutes of carboplatin administration, in which case they should be treated with appropriate supportive therapy. Myelodepression (leukopenia, neutropenia, and thrombocytopenia) is dose dependent and dose limiting, and is closely related to drug clearance.

CARMUSTINA

Trade Name/Presentation: Becenun: Ampoule containing 100 mg lyophilized powder and a proprietary diluent containing 3 mL ethyl alcohol.

Therapeutic Class: Antineoplastic, Alkylating Agent (nitrosourea).

Indication: Brain tumors, multiple myeloma, Hodgkin's lymphoma, and some solid tumors in case conventional methods fail.

Usual Dose: 200mg/m2, 1 time, every 6 weeks; 100mg/m2/day, on 2 consecutive days, every 6 weeks; or 40mg/m2/day, on 5 consecutive days, every 6 weeks. Doses vary according to the chemotherapy protocol set by the doctor. Maximum cumulative dose: 1400 mg/m$.^2$

Storage: Under refrigeration.

Route of administration/infusion time: in a peripheral vein: 1 to 2 hours, with 500mL SF in parallel.

Use a PVC-free, photosensitive line.

Reconstitution: Let the lyophilized substance and the diluent reach room temperature, reconstitute the drug with 3mL of absolute ethanol (included in the product). Then add 27mL of distilled water, resulting in a solution with 3.3mg/mL.

Stability after reconstitution: RT: 8 Hs and under refrigeration: 24 Hs.

Dilution: 250 mL of 0.9% SF or 5% SG

Stability after dilution: RT: 8 Hs and under refrigeration: 24 Hs.

Recommendations: Injection site reactions may occur during administration of BECENUN. Because of the possibility of extravasation, careful monitoring of the infusion site for possible infiltration during administration of the drug is recommended. To date, specific treatments for extravasation reactions (drug escaping from the blood vessel into the tissues adjacent to the puncture area) are not known.

Main Adverse Reactions: Infection, exfoliation in skin, swelling in face, swelling in gums, diarrhea, hair and/or hair loss, tingling, disorientation, inflammation in mucous membranes, chest discomfort, conjunctivitis, bronchospasm, alveolitis, acute respiratory distress syndrome, cytomegalovirus infection, burning sensation in skin, allergic dermatitis, eye pain, lip edema, mouth pain, jaw pain, agitation, restless leg syndrome, toothache, musculoskeletal pain, inflammation in veins, shingles, polychromasia, reticulosis, yellowish coloration of skin and mucous membranes, Staphylococcus infection, toxic nephropathy, reduced eye size, difficulty seeing close up, back pain, metabolic acidosis, muscle tension, oral discomfort, migraine, toxic rashDelayed myelodepression (decreased production of blood cells). Acute leukemia and dysplasias (abnormalities related to the development of an organ or tissue) of the bone marrow have been reported in patients after long-term treatment with nitrosureas. Nausea and vomiting Hypotension (low blood pressure), tachycardia (increased heart rate) Fever, encephalopathy, headache, shortness of breath, chest pain, breathing difficulty, interstitial lung disease, redness of the skin with or without swelling of the skin, tingling in the mouth

CYCLOPHOSPHAMIDE

Trade name/Presentation: Genuxal Injectable 200mg/cask / Genuxal Injectable 1g/cask / Genuxal 50mg/tablet.

Therapeutic Class: Antineoplastic, Alkylating agent.

Indication: Breast cancer, solid malignant tumors, lymphomas, multiple myelomas, leukemias, autoimmune diseases.

Usual Dose: Doses vary according to the chemotherapy protocol defined by the physician. Induction therapy: 40 to 50mg/Kg/day (1.5 to 1.8g/m2), IV, divided over 2 to 5 days. Maintenance therapy: 1 to 5mg/Kg/day. Oral: 10 to 15 mg/Kg daily. Injectable: every 7 to 10 weeks, 3 to 5mg/Kg, IV, twice a week. Children: 2 to 8mg/kg (60 to 250mg/m2, IV or VO divided over 6 or more days). In immunosuppressive therapy: 1 to 3mg/Kg, IV. High dosage (TMO): 60mg/Kg, for 2 days, or 6 to 7g/m2, divided by 4 days. High dosage always accompanied by the uroprotector (mesna).

Storage: Vials ampoule: TA. Tablets: Under refrigeration.

Administration route/infusion time: Apply in 5 to 10min (approximately 100mg/min). And high doses in 1 to 2h. Oral administration of cyclophosphamide should be done in the morning.

Use simple equipo.

Reconstitution: 200mg bottles: 10mL ABD; 1000mg bottles: 50mL ABD.

Stability after reconstitution: 24h Under refrigeration.

Dilution: 250 or 500 mL of 0.9% SF or 5% SG.

Stability after dilution: 24h RT or under refrigeration.

Recommendations: Only fully diluted solutions can be administered. Use uroprotectant (mesna) according to the chemotherapy protocol defined by the physician. Note: solutions containing cyclophosphamide and mesna together, even when diluted in appropriate diluents, are stable for only 24 hours TA. In oral therapy, to avoid bladder alterations, the patient should be advised to drink plenty of water on the days he takes the medication.

Main adverse reactions: Anorexia, nausea and vomiting. Significant weakening. Hair loss. Bladder alterations (with appearance of blood in the urine), which are much more frequent when the drug is taken orally.

CYPROTERONE

Trade name/Presentation: Androcur 50mg/tablet

Therapeutic Category: Antineoplastic, Hormone

Indication: In men: impulse reduction in sexual deviations, antiandrogenic treatment in inoperable prostate carcinoma. In women: severe manifestations of androgenization.

Usual Dose: Male: Impulse reduction in sexual deviations: 50mg, 2 times/day. If necessary, the dose can be increased to 100mg, 2 times/day or even 3 times/day for a short period of time. Once satisfactory clinical improvement is achieved, one should try to maintain the therapeutic effect with the lowest possible dose (Usual: 25 mg, 2 times/day). Anti-androgen treatment in inoperable prostate carcinoma: 100 mg, 2 to 3 times/day (total = 200 to 300 mg). To treat hot flashes in patients being treated with GnRH analogues or who have undergone orchiectomy: 50 to 150 mg/day, possibly up to 100 mg, 3 times/day, if necessary (total = 300 mg). Woman: The recommended dose is 100mg daily, from the 1st to the 10th day of the cycle (10 days). Additionally, a medication containing progestin-estrogen association must be used, for example, from the 1st to the 21st day of the cycle - one contraceptive tablet daily, to promote the necessary contraceptive protection and stabilize the cycle.

Storage: TA

Route of administration/infusion time: Oral.

Reconstitution: NA

Stability after reconstitution: NA

Dilution: NA

Stability after dilution: NA

Recommendations: When it is necessary to stop treatment, the dose should not be reduced abruptly, but gradually.

Main adverse reactions: Nausea, diarrhea and indigestion. Anemia. Changes in blood pressure (vasomotor), fluid retention and peripheral edema, venous thromboembolism, ischemia, congestive heart failure, pulmonary embolism, cerebrovascular accident, and electrocardiogram changes. These effects are initially seen in prostate cancer patients receiving high doses of the drug, and the risk of severe complications is greatest during the first 6 months of therapy. Sensation of breast tension and painful gynecomastia have been reported in men treated with cyproterone acetate. Vasomotor flushing with night sweats. Weight gain.

CISPLATIN

Trade Name/Presentation: Fauldcispla: Ampoule containing 50mg and vial of 100mg.

Therapeutic Class: Antineoplastic, Alkylating agent (metal salt).

Indication: Metastatic tumor of the testicle, carcinomas of the ovary, head and neck, lung, advanced bladder neoplasm.

Intravenous: 40 to 120mg/m2, IV, every 3 or 4 weeks; or 15 to 20mg/m2, IV, during 5 consecutive days, every 3 or 4 weeks; or 1mg/Kg/week, IV, for 6 weeks; or 30mg/ m^2 /week, IV. Intra-arterial: 60 to 90mg/m2, every 3 weeks; or 270mg/m2 with thiosulfate. Intraperitoneal: 50mg/m2 only D1

(in surgical cases of ovarian cancer and mesotheliioma, as single agent or associated with doxorubicin), diluted in 2L of 1.5% peritoneal dialysis solution. As a radiosensitizer: 15 to 50mg/m2, IV, up to 3 times/week (total weekly dose: 50mg/m2), concomitant to radiotherapy.

75 to 150mg/m2, intra-arterial every 2 to 5 weeks. Doses vary according to the chemotherapy protocol defined by the physician.

Storage: TA

Administration route/infusion time: It is recommended to infuse the drug at a rate not exceeding 1mg/min, or to follow the following infusion criteria: 30min - 1h: up to 60mg/m^2 ; 1h - 2h: 60mg/m^2 ; 6 - 8 h:> 60mg/m^2 . Solutions infused over a period longer than 6 hours should be protected from light (use of a light-sensitive line).

Use photoresist equipments.

Reconstitution: NA

Stability after reconstitution: 24 h TA. (Under refrigeration forms crystals).

Dilution: Dilute only in SF at minimum dilution concentration: 1mg/1mL.

Stability after dilution: 24 h TA protected from light (amber tube), do not refrigerate solutions.

Recommendations: Hyperhydration is required from 40mg/m2 onwards. To stimulate diuresis, it is common for the patient to receive 12.5 to 50g (average 37.5g) of mannitol.

Main Adverse Reactions: Nephrotoxicity, ototoxicity, anorexia, renal failure, nausea, vomiting, mucositis, myelodepression, anemia, neurotoxicity, hydroelectrolyte disturbances, hyperuricemia, ocular toxicity, hepatotoxicity, anaphylaxis.

CITARABINE

Trade Name/Presentation: Aracytin: Ampoule containing 100mg of lyophilized powder Faudcita: Ampoule containing 500mg.

Therapeutic Class: Antineoplastic, Antimetabolite (pyrimidine analog).

Indication: Leukemias and lymphomas; myelodysplastic syndrome.

Usual Dose: Intravenous: Induction therapy: 100mg/m2, every 12 hours, for 5 to 7days. Maintenance therapy: 75 to 199mg/m^2 /day for 5 days, once/week. High doses: 2 to 3g/m2, every 12 hours, for 2 to 6 days. Subcutaneous: 100mg/m2, every 12 hours, for 5 days, 1 time/month; or 10mg/m2, every 12 hours, for 15 to 21 days; or 1mg/Kg, 1 to 2 times/week. Intrathecal: 5 to 50mg/m2/day, up to 3 times/week; or 30mg/m2/day, every 4 days.

Storage: TA

Route of administration/infusion time: IV in bolus or under continuous infusion for 1 to 2 Hs (it is best under continuous infusion, as it has a short half-life). IM. IT. SC. Intraperitoneal.

Use photoresist equipments.

Reconstitution: IT: 5 mL of Nacl 0.9%. IM/SC: 2 mL of Nacl 0.9% or ABD.

Stability after reconstitution: 48 hours T.A. if reconstituted with proper diluent or immediate use if reconstituted with 0.9% SF (IT).

Dilution: For IV application: SF, SG maximum dilution concentration 60mg/mL, over 15 min, high doses do it in 2 to 3h. For IM or SC application: give preference to Aracytin 100mg. Dilute with 1 to 2 mL of SS or ABD (100 to 50mg/mL). For IT application use Aracytin 100mg (do not use another manufacturer for this administration, since the drug cannot contain preservatives). Do not dilute with the proper diluent or any other diluent with preservative: benzyl alcohol accentuates neurotoxicity.

Stability after dilution: 48 Hs TA (Aracytin) and 24 Hs (Faudcita).

Recommendations: For IT infusions: Do not consider stability. There is no antidote for cytarabine overdoses. Doses of 4.5 mg/m2 by intravenous infusion over 1 hour every 12 hours x 12 doses have caused an unacceptable increase in irreversible CNS toxicity and death. Seizures and other manifestations of neurotoxicity may occur after intrathecal administration or when high doses (greater than 3.0g/m2) are administered intravenously in patients older than 60 years or patients with poor renal function.

Main Adverse Reactions: Leukopenia, thrombocytopenia, bone marrow suppression, nausea, megaloblastosis, vomiting, anemia, diarrhea, oral inflammation or ulceration, thrombophlebitis, liver dysfunction, and fever. Much less frequently, renal dysfunction, abdominal pain, anorexia, gastrointestinal bleeding, sepsis, cellulitis at the injection site, pneumonia, neuritis or neurotoxicity, rashes, freckling, esophagitis, cutaneous and mucosal bleeding, chest pain, joint pain, sore throat, and reduced reticulocytes have been observed.

CHLORAMBUCIL

Trade Name/Presentation: Leukeran: Bottle with 25 white tablets in a dosage of 2 mg.

Therapeutic Category: Antineoplastic.

Indication: chronic lymphocytic leukemia, Hodgkin's lymphoma, non-Hodgkin's lymphoma. The indications for antineoplastic drugs are under constant review.

Usual Dose: Adults: as a starter or short cycle, 100 to 200mg/kg/day, or 3 to 6mg/m2 as a single dose or divided into several doses. Pediatric doses: 0.1 to 0.2 mg/kg as a single dose or divided into multiple doses.

Storage: Under refrigeration.

Route of administration/infusion time: Oral.

Reconstitution: NA

Stability after reconstitution: NA

Dilution: NA

Stability after dilution: NA

Recommendations: It is important to drink plenty of fluids to increase the amount of urine and facilitate the excretion of uric acid. Avoid immunizations. Gonadal suppression may occur, leading to amenorrhea and azoospermia, an effect generally related to the dose and duration of treatment. It is recommended not to use in the first trimester of pregnancy and during the lactation period. Bone marrow depressant effects may lead to an increased incidence of microbial infection, delayed healing, and bleeding gums.

Main Adverse Reactions: These are generally unavoidable and represent the pharmacological action of the drug. Frequent and dose-related are: fever, chills, or sore throat (lymphopenia, leukopenia, infection), unusual bleeding or bruising (thrombocytopenia). Less frequently: arthralgias, edema of the lower limbs, rash, dyspnea. Signs of overdose: muscle twitching, vomiting, difficulty walking, unusual excitement, and seizures.

DACARBAZINE

Trade Name/Presentation: Evodazin: Vial containing lyophilized powder in concentrations of 100 and 200 mg.

Therapeutic Category: Antineoplastic, Alkylating Agent

Indication: malignant metastatic melanoma, soft tissue sarcomas; Hodgkin's lymphoma, neuroblastoma, and renal cell carcinoma.

Usual Dose: For malignant melanoma: 150 to 250 mg/m2/day, IV, for 5 days, every 3 weeks; Hodgkin's lymphoma (in combination with other agents): 150 mg/m2/day, IV, for 5 days, every 4 weeks; or 375 mg/m2, IV, on D1 and D15, cycle repeatable every 4 weeks; (ABVD).

Storage: Under refrigeration.

Route of administration/infusion time: IV in 30 minutes. Peripheral Access: Infuse parallel SF 500mL.

Use photoresist equipments.

Reconstitution: 20mL ABD

Stability after reconstitution: Under refrigeration: 24 hours

Dilution: Dilution: 250mL to 500 mL in SF (preferred) or SG.

Stability after dilution: Concentrations of 0.4mg/mL and 0.8mg/mL in SS or GS (both protected from light - use amber tube) - 12 hours AT or 48 hours under refrigeration.

Recommendations: If there is a color change to pink or red, discard the product.

Main adverse reactions: Anorexia, nausea and vomiting. High single dose: Patients have experienced a flu-like symptom with fever at 39°C, myalgias and malaise. Alopecia, facial flushing and paresthesia.

DASATINIBE

Trade name/Presentation: Sprycel 50mg/coated tablet.

Therapeutic Class: Antineoplastic, Tyrosine Kinase Inhibitor.

Indication: Treatment of chronic myeloid leukemia in adults who are not benefiting from or have intolerance to prior therapy, including imatinib mesylate. Treatment of Philadelphia chromosome-positive acute lymphoblastic leukemia in adults who are not benefiting from or have intolerance to prior therapy.

Usual Dose: Chronic myeloid leukemia (Chronic phase): 100mg VO once a day. Chronic myeloid leukemia (Accelerated Phase) and Philadelphia chromosome-positive acute lymphoblastic leukemia: 140mg VO once daily.

Storage: TA.

Route of administration/infusion time: Oral.

Reconstitution: NA.

Stability after reconstitution: NA.

Dilution: NA.

Stability after dilution: NA.

Recommendations: Administer once daily (morning or evening), at the same time each day, with or without food. The tablets should be swallowed whole with the help of a glass of water and should not be chewed, broken or crushed.

Major Adverse Reactions: myelosuppression, fluid retention, diarrhea, headache, dyspnea, skin rash, fatigue, nausea, and hemorrhage. pleural effusion, gastrointestinal bleeding, febrile neutropenia, dyspnea, pneumonia, pyrexia diarrhea, infection, congestive heart failure/heart failure, pericardial effusion, and Central Nervous System hemorrhage.

DAUNORRUBICIN

Trade name/Presentation: Daunoblastine injectable 20mg/flask.

Therapeutic Category: Antineoplastic, Antibiotic.

Indication: acute leukemias (lymphocytic, myelocytic, erythrocytic), lymphomas, neuroblastoma, chronic myeloid leukemia, Ewing's sarcoma, Wilms' tumor.

Usual Dose: 30 to 60mg/m2/day, IV, for 3 days, every 3 to 4 weeks; or 0.8 to 1.0mg/Kg/day, IV, for 3 to 6 days, every 3 to 4 weeks; or in combination with cytarabine: 45 mg/m2/day, IV (30 mg/m2/day if patient is 60 years or older), for 3 days in the 1st cycle and 2 days in subsequent cycles. Children: 25 to 45 mg/m2/day, IV, for 3 days; or 25 mg/m2/week, IV, in combination with vincristine and prednisone.

Storage: TA

Administration route/infusion time: 30 to 45 minutes. Peripheral access: Infuse parallel 250mL SF.

Simple equipment.

Reconstitution: ABD 10 mL.

Stability after reconstitution: RT: 24 Hours. Under refrigeration: 48 Hours.

Dilution: 0.9% SF or 5% SGI: 100 mL.

Stability after dilution: RT: 24 Hours.

Recommendations: this drug contains sugar, so it should be used with caution in diabetics.

Main adverse reactions: Nausea; vomiting; diarrhea (increase in the number and amount of feces eliminated daily), esophagitis (inflammation of the esophagus), mucositis/stomatitis (inflammation of the mucosa of the mouth that can cause pain or burning sensation, erythema (redness), erosion-ulceration, bleeding, infections); irreversible hair loss; cellulitis; skin peeling. infection, sepsis/septicemia (generalized infection). Bone marrow failure (change in the function of the marrow that produces blood), granulocytopenia (decrease in the number of platelets, clotting cells), leukopenia (decrease in the number of white blood cells in the blood), neutropenia (decrease in the number of neutrophils in the blood), thrombocytopenia (decrease in the number of platelets), and anemia (decrease in the number of red blood cells: RBCs). cardiomyopathy (impaired function of the heart muscle leading to improper heart function) clinically manifested by dyspnea (shortness of breath), cyanosis (blue-purple coloration of the skin due to lack of oxygen), peripheral cardiac edema (swelling), hepatomegaly (enlargement of the liver), ascites (accumulation of fluid within the abdominal cavity), pleural effusion (presence of fluid between the membranes that protect the heart), and congestive heart failure (inability of the heart to pump an adequate amount of blood). Hemorrhage (bleeding). Alopecia (hair loss), erythema (redness), rash (redness of the skin).

DOCETAXEL

Trade name/Presentation: Docetaxel/Docelibbs: 20 and 80 mg. Taxotere: 20 and 80 mg.

Therapeutic Class: Antineoplastic, Antimicrotubule agent.

Indication: Breast cancer, lung cancer, ovarian cancer, head and neck cancer, prostate cancer, pancreatic cancer, and soft tissue sarcomas.

Usual Dose: 50 to 100 mg/m^2 , every 3 weeks.

Storage: Under refrigeration.

Route of administration/infusion time: IV: 1 hour.

Simple equipment.

Reconstitution: Leave the vial 5 minutes at room temperature. Reconstitute with the diluent that comes with the product. Do not shake. Just invert the vial repeatedly, obtaining a homogeneous solution of final concentration 10mg/ml.

Stability after reconstitution: Immediate use.

Dilution: 250 mL of SF 0.9% or SG 5%. Dose > 200 mg: a higher volume of solution should be used for dilution, aiming not to exceed a concentration of 0.74 mg/ mL of docetaxel.

Stability after dilution: RT: 4h including 1h of infusion.

Recommendations: Careful monitoring of vital functions during infusion.

Main Adverse Reactions: Vasodilatation, edema. Alopecia, nail changes, pruritus, rash, Stevens-Johnson syndrome and toxic epidermal necrolysis, diarrhea, nausea, stomatitis, vomiting and colitis, anemia, leukopenia, neutropenia and thrombocytopenia, asthenia, eneuropathy, interstitial pneumonia and pulmonary embolism, anaphylaxis, amenorrhea, hepatotoxicity, renal failure, fever.

DOXORRUBICIN

Trade Name/Presentation: Fauldoxo: 50 mg/25 mL and 10 mg/ 5 mL.

Therapeutic Category: Antineoplastic, Antibiotic.

Indication: breast, lung, bladder, liver, thyroid, and ovarian carcinomas; sarcomas; lymphomas; acute lymphoid leukemia; acute myeloid leukemia, Wilms' tumor.

Usual Dose: The dose varies according to the chemotherapy protocol adopted by the doctor, as a single agent (60 to 70mg/m2 every 3 weeks) or in combination with other drugs (25 to 50mg/m2 every 3 weeks). The cumulative dose should not exceed 550mg/m2.

Storage: Under refrigeration.

Route of administration/infusion time: IV/Intra-arterial/Intra-vesical. IV: Infuse 20-30 min in 100 mL 0.9% saline solution.

Photosensitive equipment.

Reconstitution: Ready to use.

Stability after reconstitution: Under refrigeration: 48 Hs.

Dilution: 100 mL SF 0.9%.

Stability after dilution: RT: 24 Hs.

Recommendation: The limiting cumulative intravenous dose, regardless of dosing plan, is 550 mg/m^2 . It may turn your urine red for a day or two after treatment. This type of medicine decreases the number of some types of blood cells in your body, so you may bleed or get infections more easily. It is recommended that you avoid contact with sick people; wash your hands frequently; stay away from dangerous situations where you might get hurt, such as playing sports and using sharp objects; brush your teeth and floss gently.

Main adverse reactions: Congestive heart failure (decreased heart function); arrhythmias; alopecia (hair loss); nausea; vomiting; stomatitis; esophagitis; diarrhea; dehydration; facial flushing; reddish coloration of urine.

ETHOPOSITE

Trade Name/Presentation: Posidon/Eunades: Ampoule bottle: 100mg - 20mg/mL (5mL bottle).

Vepesid 50mg/capsule.

Therapeutic Class: Antineoplastic, semisynthetic derivative of podophyllotoxin.

Indication: testicular, lung, Hodgkin and non-Hodgkin lymphomas, acute non-lymphocytic leukemia, and brain tumors.

Usual Dose: *Injectable:* 35 to 100mg/m2/day, IV, for 3 to 5 days, every 3 to 4 weeks; or 125 to 140mg/m2/day, IV, on days 1,3 and 5, every 3 to 5 weeks; or 120mg/m2/day, IV, for 3 days, every 3 weeks; or 200 to 250mg/m2/week. High-dose: 750 to 2400mg/m2 or 400 to 800mg/m2/day, for 3 days, for 1 or 2 courses. *Oral:* double the injectable dose, same regimen; or 50mg/m2/day, for 21 days, followed by 1 to 2 weeks rest. Dose varies according to the chemotherapy protocol adopted by the physician.

Storage: TA

Route of administration/infusion time: Slow IV (usually within a 30 to 60 minute period) as hypotension has been reported as a possible side effect of rapid IV injection. Tablets: VO: Ingest on an empty stomach.

Simple equipment.

Reconstitution: Bottle: Ready to use.

Stability after reconstitution: T.A: 16 hours.

Dilution: 0.9% SF or 5% SG, concentration 0.2 to 0.4mg/mL.

Stability after dilution: Under refrigeration: 24h.

Recommendations: Etoposide should not be administered by rapid Intravenous infusion. When necessary, the injectable solution may be used orally if mixed with orange juice or lemonade, in a concentration of 0.4mg/mL. Use the mixture within 3 hours. The most significant toxicity associated with etoposide therapy is dose-limiting bone marrow depression. There is the possibility of an anaphylactic reaction manifesting as chills, fever, tachycardia, bronchospasm, dyspnea, and hypotension. Treatment is symptomatic. The infusion should be stopped immediately, followed by administration of pressor agents, corticosteroids, antihistamines, or volume expanders, at the physician's discretion.

Main Adverse Reactions: Myelosuppression, with granulocyte nadir occurring in 7 to 14 days and platelet nadir occurring in 9 to 16 days after drug administration. Bone marrow recovery occurs in approximately 20 days. The occurrence of acute leukemia, with or without a pre-leukocytic phase, has been reported in a few cases with associated therapy. Reversible leukopenia, thrombocytopenia and anemia. Nausea and vomiting, which may be controlled with antiemetic therapy. Anorexia, diarrhea and stomatitis may also occur. Hypotension may occur with very rapid I.V. injection; it is not associated with cardiac toxicity or electrocardiographic alterations. Anaphylactic type reactions can occur, characterized by fever, tachycardia, hypertension, bronchospasm, dyspnea and/or hypotension. These reactions, however, can be fatal. Coughing, diaphoresis, cyanosis, laryngospasm, back pain and/or loss of consciousness, and hypersensitivity associated with apnea sometimes occur. Rare cases of bronchopulmonary anaphylaxis (2% of cases). Reversible alopecia. Peripheral paresthesias, fever, pigmentation, abdominal pain, constipation, dysphagia, transient cortical blindness and optic neuritis, liver toxicity and acidosis (in patients receiving higher than recommended doses), peripheral neurotoxicity.

FILGRASTIN

Trade Name/Presentation: Filgrastin: Ampoule bottle;, Granulokine: Filled syringe: Contains 1 mL corresponding to 30 million units (300 mcg).

Therapeutic Class: Hematopoietic Growth Factor, Granulocyte Colony Stimulating Factor.

Indication: Reduction in the duration of neutropenia and incidence of febrile neutropenia in patients with non-myeloablative neoplasms treated with established cytotoxic chemotherapy; reduction in the duration of neutropenia and its clinical sequelae in patients undergoing myeloablative therapy followed by bone marrow transplantation; mobilization of peripheral progenitor cells (PBPC).

Usual Dose: Adults and Children: Cancer chemotherapy: 5mcg/kg/ kg/day, SC or IV, 24h after last dose of chemotherapy, and continuing until neutrophil count reaches desired level (>1,000/mm3), increase to 15mcg/kg/dose, SC or IV, 1 time/day, if desired effect is not achieved within 1 week. BMT: 10mcg/kg/day, IV, within 24h after bone marrow infusion.

Storage: Under refrigeration.

Route of administration/infusion time: IV daily in SG 5% during 30 minutes or 24 Hs. SC daily up to 14 days.

Reconstitution: Ready to use.

Stability after reconstitution: NA.

Dilution: Recommended dilution: dilute each vial with 20mL of SG5% for a final Concentration = 15mcg/mL. For concentrations greater than 5mcg/mL and less than 15mcg/mL, it is necessary to add 2mg of Human Albumin 20% (0.01mL) for each mL of solution. For example, for a final injection volume of 40mL, 0.4mL of a 20% Human Albumin solution should be added. It is not recommended that the final solution concentration be less than 5mcg/mL.

Stability after dilution: 24 Hs under refrigeration.

Recommendations: The use of Fligrastima is not recommended in cases of renal and hepatic insufficiency.

Main Adverse Reactions: Administration at the recommended doses is often associated with musculoskeletal pain specifically in bone marrow. Generally mild or moderate, but occasionally severe and is usually controlled with classical analgesics. Urinary abnormalities (predominantly mild or moderate dysuria). Transient hypotension, not requiring clinical treatment, has occasionally been reported. Adverse events reported with equal frequency in patients treated with figrastim/chemotherapy and placebo/chemotherapy included nausea and vomiting, alopecia, diarrhea, fatigue, anorexia, mucositis, headache, cough, skin rash, chest pain, generalized weakness, sore throat, constipation, and nonspecific pain. Vascular disorders (e.g., veno-occlusive disease and fluid volume disturbances) have occasionally been reported in patients undergoing high-dose chemotherapy post autologous bone marrow transplantation.

FLUDARABINE

Trade Name/Presentation: Fludara: Vials of 50 mg lyophilized powder.

Therapeutic Class: Antineoplastic, Antimetabolite (purine analog).

Indication: Leukemias and Lymphomas.

Usual Dose: 25 mg/m2/day, IV, for 5 consecutive days, every 28 days.

Storage: TA.

Route of administration/infusion time: IV 30 minutes.

Simple equipment.

Reconstitution: Reconstitute each vial with 2mL of ABD, resulting in 25 mg/mL.

Stability after reconstitution: 8 Hs TA.

Dilution: SF 0.9% 100 mL.

Stability after dilution: Immediate use.

Recommendations: This drug is contraindicated for use by patients with severe kidney problems (creatinine clearance < 30 mL/min).

Main adverse reactions: infections (some serious infections): infections due to depression of the immune system (opportunistic infections); infections of the lungs (pneumonia); reduced number of platelets (thrombocytopenia) with the possibility of bruising and bleeding; reduced number of white blood cells (neutropenia); reduced number of red blood cells (anemia);

cough; vomiting, diarrhea, feeling sick (nausea); fever; feeling tired (fatigue); weakness. bone marrow depression (myelosuppression); severe appetite loss leading to weight loss (anorexia); numbness or weakness in the limbs (peripheral neuropathy; blurred vision; inflammation of the inside of the mouth (stomatitis); skin rashes; chills; generally feeling unwell; swelling due to excessive fluid retention (edema); inflammation of the mucous membranes of the digestive system from the mouth to the anus (mucositis).

FLUORURACIL

Trade Name/Presentation: Fluorouracil: Ampoule bottle: 500mg - 50mg/mL (10mL ampoule bottle) and 2500 mg - 50 mg/mL (50mL ampoule bottle).

Therapeutic Class: Antineoplastic, Antimetabolite (pyrimidine analog).

Indication: Malignant tumors of the lung, breast, colon and rectum, gastric, liver, head and neck, uterine, ovary and bladder carcinomas.

Usual Dose: Administer 7 to 12 mg per kg body weight for 4 days. Take a 3-day break, and then administer 7 to 10 mg per body weight daily for 2 weeks.

Storage: TA.

Route of administration/infusion time: Can be given as an infusion or intravenous injection. **Plain IV Sets for infusions under 1 hour and light-sensitive sets for infusions over 1 hour.**

Reconstitution: Ready to use.

Stability after reconstitution: RT: 24 Hs.

Dilution: 0.9% SF.

Stability after dilution: RT: 48 Hs.

Recommendations: It is not recommended to use the same vein for consecutive applications. Overdosage: The possibility of overdosage with fluorouracil is uncommon in view of the mode of administration, although early manifestations could be nausea, vomiting, diarrhea, gastrointestinal ulceration and bleeding, bone marrow depression (including thrombocytopenia, leukopenia, and agranulocytosis). There is no specific antidote therapy. Patients who have been exposed to fluorouracil overdose should be monitored hematologically for at least 4 weeks.

Major Adverse Reactions: Adverse effects associated with prolonged use of arterial catheterization include: arterial ischemia, thrombosis, catheter site bleeding, catheter obstruction, embolism, fibrosis, catheter site infection, abscess, and thrombophlebitis. The following side effects have been grouped based on clinical significance. Leukopenia is the most common toxic effect. Nausea, vomiting, anorexia, dermatitis, pigmentation, alopecia, nail loss, stomatitis, diarrhea, gastrointestinal ulceration, bleeding, ataxia, fever, hemorrhage, thrombocytopenia. The toxic effects can be severe and sometimes fatal. Reducing the speed of injection to a slow infusion for 2 to 8 hours may reduce toxicity, but this may be less effective than rapid injection of the drug. Leukopenia may not be significant until stomatitis occurs. The drop in WBC count is greatest between day 9 and day 20, returning to normal by day 30. Thrombocytopenia is usually maximum in 7 to 17 days after the first dose.

FULVESTRANTO

Trade Name/Presentation: Faslodex Injectable - 250mg/syringe 5mL.

Therapeutic Class: Antineoplastic, antiestrogen.

Indication: Treatment for postmenopausal women of any age with locally advanced or metastatic breast cancer.

Usual Dose: 250 mg, IM in the gluteal region, at intervals of one month.

Storage: Under refrigeration.

Route of administration/infusion time:

Reconstitution: The solution comes ready to use, in a filled syringe, just remove the air and connect the needle at the time of administration.

Stability after reconstitution: NA

Dilution: NA

Stability after dilution: NA

Recommendations: Caution should be exercised with the use of FASLODEX in patients with moderate to severe hepatic insufficiency, in whom clearance may be altered. Caution should be exercised before treating patients who have creatinine clearance less than 30 ml/min. Caution should be exercised before treating patients with bleeding, thrombocytopenia, or those taking anticoagulants due to the route of administration. Effects on ability to drive vehicles and operate machinery: FASLODEX is unlikely to interfere with the ability to drive vehicles and operate machinery. However, during treatment with FASLODEX, asthenia has been reported, and patients with this symptom should be carefully observed.

Main adverse reactions: Nausea; vomiting; constipation; diarrhea; stomach pain; headache; fatigue; hot flushes; pharyngitis.

GENCITABINE

Trade Name/Presentation: Gemzar/Gemcit: Vials containing lyophilized powder in concentrations of 200 and 1000 mg.

Therapeutic Class: Antineoplastic, Antimetabolite.

Indication: Cancer of the bladder, pancreas, lung, breast, ovary, and testicle; pancreatic adenocarcinoma, lymphomas, and sarcomas.

Usual Dose: 1000mg/m2, once a week for 7 weeks, followed by 1 week break, subsequent applications weekly for 3 weeks, followed by 1 week break

Storage: TA

Route of administration/infusion time: IV 30min. Increased infusion rate at a fixed dose of 10mg/ m^2 /min is associated with a higher incidence of side effects, but greater clinical benefit.

Simple equipment.

Reconstitution: 200mg vials: 5 mL of 0.9% SF and 1g vials with 25mL, resulting in a concentration of 40mg/mL.

Stability after reconstitution: RT: 24 Hs.

Dilution: SF 0.9% 500mL, at a maximum concentration of 0.1mg/mL.

Stability after dilution: RT: 24 Hs.

Recommendations: Do not refrigerate the medication.

Main adverse reactions: Peripheral edema. Alopecia and skin rash. Constipation, diarrhea, nausea, vomiting and stomatitis. Anemia, leukopenia, neutropenia, thrombocytopenia. Paresthesia and sensory neuropathy. Dyspnea. Fatigue, fever, and pain Infarction and heart failure. Hypersensitivity and anaphylaxis.

GOSSERRELINA

Trade Name/Presentation: Zoladex Injectable 3.6mg/syringe

Zoladex LA injectable 10.8mg/syringe

Therapeutic Category: Antineoplastic, Hormone. Gonadotropin-releasing hormone agonist.

Indication: control of prostate and breast cancer amenable to hormonal manipulation (palliative treatment); control of endometriosis; uterine leiomyoma; decrease in endometrial thickness.

Usual Dose: Syringes: 3.6 mg every 28 days, for 3 months. Syringes: 10.8 mg every 3 months.

Storage: Under refrigeration.

Route of administration/infusion time: SC injection into the upper abdominal wall.

Reconstitution: NA.

Stability after reconstitution: NA.

Dilution: NA.

Stability after dilution: NA.

Recommendations: After discontinuation of therapy with Zoladex LA 10.8 mg, the time to return to menstruation may be prolonged in some patients. The use of Zoladex may cause increased cervical resistance and caution should be taken when dilating the cervix. To date, there are no clinical data on the efficacy of treating benign gynecological conditions with Zoladex for periods longer than 6 months. It is not indicated for children, as the safety and efficacy of gosserrelin have not been established in this group of patients. Zoladex 3.6 mg should only be administered as part of a regimen for assisted reproduction, under the supervision of a specialist experienced in this field. As with other LHRH agonists, there are some reports of Ovarian Hyperstimulation Syndrome (OHS) associated with the use of Zoladex 3.6 mg in combination with gonadotropins. The stimulation cycle should be carefully monitored to identify patients at risk of developing this syndrome. Human gonadotrophin (hCG) should be blocked if appropriate. Caution is recommended when using Zoladex 3.6 mg in assisted reproduction regimens in patients with Polycystic Ovary Syndrome (PCOS), as there may be increased recruitment of follicles. Zoladex should not be used during pregnancy, as there is a theoretical risk of miscarriage or fetal abnormality if LHRH agonists are used during pregnancy. Potentially fertile women should be carefully screened prior to initiation of treatment to exclude pregnancy. Non-hormonal contraceptive methods should be used during treatment until menstruation returns. Only after menstruation has returned can hormonal contraceptive methods be used. Pregnancy must be excluded before Zoladex 3.6 mg is used for assisted fertilization. When employed for this purpose, there is no clinical evidence to suggest a causal association between Zoladex 3.6 mg and any subsequent abnormality of oocyte development or pregnancy and delivery. The use of Zoladex during the breastfeeding period is contraindicated. Administration of Zoladex in therapeutic doses results in suppression of the pituitary-gonadal system. Diagnostic tests of gonadotropic and gonadal pituitary function performed during treatment with Zoladex and until menstrual flow resumes may show altered results due to its suppressive effect. Normal function is usually restored within 12 weeks after discontinuation of treatment.

Main Adverse Reactions: Most common are headache, emotional lability, depression, bone pain, insomnia, hot flashes, sexual dysfunction, decreased libido, impotence, lower urinary tract symptoms, diaphoresis. Less common are palpitation, tachycardia, edema, CHF, angina, hypertension, AMI; anorexia, nausea, vomiting, diarrhea, abdominal pain, dyspepsia, ulcer; anemia, bleeding; infections.

HYDROXYURE

Commercial Name/Presentation: Hydrea 500mg/capsule.

Therapeutic Class: Antineoplastic, Antimetabolite.

Indication: treatment of melanoma, refractory chronic myelocytic leukemia, relapsed and refractory metastatic ovarian cancer.

Usual Dose: Solid tumors: Intermittent therapy: 80mg/Kg VO every 3 days. Continuous therapy: 20-30mg/Kg/day VO. Resistant Chronic Myelocytic Leukemia: 20 30mg/Kg/day VO.

Storage: TA.

Route of administration/Infusion time: The capsules should be swallowed whole, at the same time every day.

Reconstitution: NA.

Stability after reconstitution: NA.

Dilution: NA.

Stability after dilution: NA.

Recommendations: Patients should be cautioned to maintain an adequate fluid intake. It is contraindicated in patients who have blood disorders (reduced levels of red and white blood cells and/or platelets).

Main Adverse Reactions: The occurrence of adverse reactions such as gastrointestinal symptoms (stomatitis, loss of appetite, nausea, vomiting, diarrhea and constipation) and skin reactions (maculopapular rash and redness of the face) should be reported to the attending physician. Treatment with this drug should always be done under careful medical supervision and periodic blood tests should be performed in order to detect early any hematological changes, such as anemia, decrease in the number of white blood cells or platelets.

<h1 style="text-align:center">IFOSFAMIDE</h1>

Trade Name/Presentation: Evolox/Holoxane: Ampoule containing 1000 mg lyophilized powder.

Therapeutic Class: Antineoplastic, Alkylating agent.

Indication: testicular tumor, ovarian carcinoma, breast, lung, stomach, endometrium, kidney and pancreas, soft tissue sarcoma, osteosarcoma, malignant lymphomas, and acute leukemias.

Usual Dose: Children: 1200mg to 1800mg/m^2 /day, for 3-5 days, every 21-28 days; 5000mg/m^2 /day, IV, once, every 21-28 days. Adults: 700 to 2000mg/m^2 /day, IV, for 5 days every 21-28 days; 2.5 to 4g/m^2 /day, IV, for 2-3 days every 21-28 days; 5 to 6g/m^2 /day (maximum 10g), in a 24-hour infusion, every 21-28 days.

Storage: TA

Route of administration/infusion time: IV: Should not be less than 30 minutes and is usually done in 1-2 hours, or also in continuous infusion.

Simple equipment.

Reconstitution: ABD 25 mL. Wait 30 to 60 seconds and then shake the vial with vigorous movements.

Stability after reconstitution: Under refrigeration: 24hs.

Dilution: 0.9% SF, 5% SG, or Ringer-lactate, in concentrations from 0.6 to 20mg/mL.

Stability after dilution: RT: 24 Hs.

Recommendations: Use mesna 20% of the total IV dose at time 0, 4 hours and 8 hours, for prevention of bleeding cystitis.

Main adverse reactions: Alopecia. Nausea and vomiting. Myelosuppression. Neurotoxicity. Nephrotoxicity.

<h1 style="text-align:center">IMATINIBE</h1>

Trade name/Presentation: Gleevec 100mg/tablet

Gleevec 400mg/tablet

Therapeutic Class: Antineoplastic, tyrosine kinase inhibitor.

Indication: Treatment of adult patients with newly diagnosed Philadelphia chromosome positive chronic myeloid leukemia; adult patients with newly diagnosed Philadelphia chromosome positive acute lymphoblastic leukemia; and adult patients with gastrointestinal stromal tumors that are non-resectable and/or metastatic.

Usual Dose: Treatment of chronic myeloid leukemia (chronic phase): 400mg/day, Treatment of chronic myeloid leukemia (accelerated phase or blastic crisis): 600mg/day. Treatment of acute lymphoblastic leukemia: 600mg/day. Treatment of gastrointestinal stomach tumors: 400mg/day.

Storage: TA.

Route of administration/infusion time: VO.

Reconstitution: NA.

Stability after reconstitution: NA.

Dilution: NA.

Stability after dilution: NA.

Recommendations: The tablets should be swallowed whole with the aid of a glass of water.

Major Adverse Reactions: Rapid weight gain, swelling of extremities (calves, ankles), generalized swelling such as puffiness of face (signs of water retention); Weakness, spontaneous bleeding or bruising, frequent infections with signs such as fever, chills, sore throat, mouth ulcers (signs of low blood cell levels). Pallor, tiredness, shortness of breath, dark urine (signs of low red blood cell levels); Sudden weakening of vision, blurred vision, visible bleeding in the white of the eye; Tightness or pain in the chest, irregular heartbeat (signs of heart problems); Nausea, diarrhea, vomiting, abdominal pain, fever (signs of inflammatory bowel disease); Rash (rash), redness of the skin, blistering of the lips, eyes, skin, or mouth, peeling of the skin, fever, red or purple spots on the skin, itching, burning, postural rash (signs of skin disorders); Pain in the hips or difficulty walking; Inflammation and acute redness of the skin caused by an infection (sign of cellulitis); Severe headache, weakness or paralysis of limbs or face, difficulty speaking, sudden loss of consciousness, or seizures (signs of nervous system disorders); Hearing impairment; Dizziness, lightheadedness, or fainting; Cold or numb fingers or toes (signs of Raynaud's syndrome); Severe abdominal pain, vomiting with blood, blood in stools or urine, or dark stools Nausea, loss of appetite, dark urine or yellowing of the skin or eyes (signs of liver problems); Decreased amount of urine, thirst; Swelling and pain in some part of the body; Cough, difficulty breathing, painful breathing; Muscle weakness, muscle spasms, abnormal heart rhythm (signs of changes in the blood potassium level); Bruising (with local bruising); Gastric pain, nausea. Muscle spasm, fever, reddish-brown urine, pain or weakness in muscles (signs of muscle disorders) Pelvic pain sometimes accompanied by nausea and vomiting, unexpected vaginal bleeding, dizziness, fainting, decreased blood pressure (signs of gynecological disorder) Headache; Nausea, diarrhea, vomiting, indigestion, abdominal pain; Pruritus, redness, burning, rash (rash); Muscle cramps, muscle and bone pain, joint pain; Swelling of the eyelids or around the eye; Fatigue; Weight gain. Insomnia; Dizziness; Tingling, pain, or numbness in the hands, feet, legs, or around the hip; Changes in taste; Decreased skin sensitivity; Itching and discharge from the eye, redness and swelling (conjunctivitis), increased tear production, dry eye; Flushing; Nasal bleeding; Dry mouth; Abdominal bloating, flatulence, constipation, heartburn, nausea, and stomach pain (sign of gastritis); Abnormal results on liver function lab tests; Dry skin; Itching; Unusual thinning or hair loss; Night sweats; Increased skin sensitivity to the sun (sign of photosensitivity); Swelling of joints; Chills; Weight loss; Loss of appetite; Ulceration in the mouth. Redness and/or swelling on the palms of the hands and soles of the feet, which may be accompanied by tingling and burning.

IRINOTECAN

Commercial Name/Presentation: Evoterin: Ampoule with 100mg (20mg/mL- 5mL bottle).

Therapeutic Class: Antineoplastic, Topoisomerase I inhibitor.

Indication: Metastatic carcinoma of the colon and rectum, pancreas, lung, stomach, and ovary.

Usual Dose: 125mg/m2 weekly, for 4 weeks, followed by rest for 2 weeks. 200 to 350mg/m2, every 3-4 weeks; 40mg/m2/day, for 5 days, every 4 weeks; 60mg/m2/week, for 3 weeks (D1, D8, D15) every 4 weeks.

Storage: TA.

Route of administration/infusion time: IV, over 90 minutes.

Photoresist Equipo.

Reconstitution: Ready to use.

Stability after reconstitution: Under refrigeration: 24 Hs.

Dilution: SG 5% or SF 0.9% 500 mL.

Stability after dilution: RT: 06 Hs and under refrigeration: 24 Hs in SG 5%.

Recommendations: When the patient presents with early diarrhea, use in subsequent cycles atropine at a dose of 0.25 to 1mg.

Main Adverse Reactions: late diarrhea, nausea, vomiting, early diarrhea, abdominal pain/cramps, anorexia, stomatitis leukopenia, anemia, neutropenia, asthenia, fever weight loss, dehydration, alopecia, thromboembolic events (Include angina pectoris, arterial thrombosis, cerebral infarction, stroke, deep thrombophlebitis, lower extremity embolism, cardiac arrest, myocardial infarction, myocardial ischemia, peripheral vascular disorder, pulmonary embolism, sudden death, thrombophlebitis, thrombosis, vascular disorder).

L-ASPARAGINASE

Trade Name/Presentation: Elspar Injectable 10,000IU/flask.

Therapeutic Class: Antineoplastic, Enzyme (derived from Escherichia coli).

Indication: acute lymphocytic leukemia.

Usual Dose: Adults: 6,000UI to 10,000UI/day IM, 9-12 times, every 1 or 3 days, or 20,000UI/m^2 , 3 times/week. Children: 1000 IUI/Kg/day, IV or IM, for 10 successive days, or 6,000 IUI/m^2 , every 3 days. The dose may vary according to the chemotherapy protocol defined by the physician. Dose for intradermal testing: 2 IUI.

Storage: Under refrigeration.

Route of administration/infusion time: IM or IV. IV: At least 30 minutes.

Reconstitution: IM: 2 mL of ABD or 0.9% saline solution; IV: 5 mL of ABD or 0.9% saline solution.

Stability after reconstitution: Under refrigeration: 8 Hs.

Dilution: 50mL to 100mL of 0.9% SF or 5% SG

Stability after dilution: Under refrigeration: 8 Hs.

Recommendations: IM route preferred. Avoid excessive agitation of the vial. Allergic reactions to L- asparaginase are frequent and may occur in the initial cycle of therapy. These reactions are not entirely predictable on the basis of the intradermal test. Perform intradermal testing if patient is being treated for the first time: Because of the occurrence of allergic reactions, intradermal testing should be performed before the initial administration of ELSPAR® and when ELSPAR® is given after the interval of one week or more between doses. The solution for intradermal testing can be prepared as follows: **reconstitute the contents of a 10,000 Ul ampoule with 5 mL of diluent. Take 0.1 mL of this solution (2000 IU/mL) and place it in another ampoule containing 9.9 mL of diluent, thus having an**

intradermal test solution of approximately 20.0 UI/mL. Use 0.1 mL of this solution (plus or minus 2.0 UI) for the intradermal test.

The test site should be observed for at least one hour until either papule or erythema appears, either of which indicates a positive reaction. An allergic reaction, even to an intradermal test dose, may occur rarely in certain sensitized individuals. A negative intradermal test does not rule out the possibility of developing allergic reactions.

The maximum volume at each injection site should be 2 mL. If the required volume is greater than 2 mL, then it should be injected at two different sites.

Main Adverse Reactions: Allergic reactions including skin rashes, urticaria, arthralgia, dyspnea, and acute anaphylaxis.

LEUPRORRELINA

Trade Name/Presentation: Lectrun: Ampoules containing lyophilized powder in concentrations of 3.75 mg and 7.5 mg + proper diluent.

Therapeutic Category: Gonadotropic Hormones.

Indication: treatment of advanced prostate cancer, as an alternative to orchiectomy or estrogen administration. Breast cancer. Endometriosis. Uterine Fibroma. Uterine leiomyosarcoma. Premature puberty.

Usual Dose: 3.75 or 7.5 mg monthly.

Storage: TA.

Route of administration/infusion time: IM.

Reconstitution: Take 1.5 mL of the proper diluent that comes in the kit, place in the vial containing the lyophilized powder, shake the vial until all powder is reconstituted, withdraw the 1.5 mL in the syringe.

Stability after reconstitution: NA.

Dilution: NA.

Stability after dilution: NA.

Recommendations: In most patients, testosterone levels increased above baseline for the first week, thereafter declining to baseline or lower levels by the end of the second week of treatment. This transient increase in hormone levels was occasionally associated with a temporary worsening of signs and symptoms. Special attention should be devoted to patients with vertebral metastases and/or urinary obstruction or hematuria, as a potential worsening of signs and symptoms early in the course of treatment may lead to neurological problems, such as weakness and/or paresthesia of the lower limbs, or worsening of urinary symptoms.

Main adverse reactions: People in whom the tumor has reached the spinal bones (vertebrae) and/or who are unable to urinate due to obstruction by the tumor: Weakness and/or loss of feeling in the lower limbs or worsening of urinary symptoms; Weakness, generalized pain, headache, injection site reaction; Heat waves, increased sweating; Gastrointestinal changes (stomach and intestines); Joint problems; Dizziness, lightheadedness, insomnia, sleep changes, neuromuscular changes; Respiratory changes; Skin reactions; Testicular atrophy, urinary changes; Changes in laboratory tests.

LOMUSTINA

Trade Name/Presentation: Citostal: Capsules in concentrations of 10 and 40mg.

Therapeutic Class: Antineoplastic, Alkylating agent.

Indication: Palliative therapy in association with other treatment modalities or in established combinations with other antineoplastic agents in primary or metastatic brain tumors, in patients who have already received appropriate surgical and/or radiotherapeutic treatment; Hodgkin's disease, as secondary therapy; and other tumors when conventional methods have failed.

Usual Dose: 130mg/m² as a single dose every 6 weeks. Subsequent doses to the initial dose should be adjusted according to the patient's hematological response to the previous dose.

Storage: TA.

Route of administration/infusion time: VO.

Reconstitution: NA.

Stability after reconstitution: NA.

Dilution: NA.

Stability after dilution: NA.

Recommendations: Impaired spinal cord function: reduce dose to 100mg/m² as a single dose every 6 weeks. The drug should be administered fasting, maintained for 2 hours after drug administration.

Main Adverse Reactions: Fever, chills, sore throat, unusual bleeding or bruising, difficulty breathing, dry cough, swelling of the feet or legs, mental confusion, or yellowing of the eyes and skin. Nausea and vomiting usually last less than 24 hours, however loss of appetite can last several days.

MELFALAN

Trade name/Presentation: Alkeran 2mg/tablet

Therapeutic Class: Antineoplastic, Alkylating Agent (Mechlorethamine derivative)

Indication: Multiple myeloma, advanced breast and ovarian cancer, sarcomas, melanoma, prostate, testicular and lung cancer, chronic myeloid leukemia and bone marrow transplant conditioning protocols. Intra-arterial for limb perfusion in melanoma.

Usual Dose: The recommended dose of Alkeran depends on several factors, including the indication for use, the severity of the disease, co-morbid conditions of the patient, the patient's hematologic status and the route of administration. Therefore, as each case requires a clinical decision based on several factors, recommendations for maximum daily dosage cannot be provided. **Multiple myeloma:** A typical oral dosing regimen is 0.15 mg/kg body weight/day, in divided doses over four days, repeated at 6-week intervals. **Advanced ovarian adenocarcinoma:** A typical oral regimen is 0.2 mg/kg body weight/day for 5 days. This regimen is repeated every 4 to 8 weeks, or as soon as peripheral blood counts are recovered. **Breast cancer:** Alkeran has been administered orally at a dose of 0.15 mg/kg body weight or 6 mg/ m^2 body surface area/day for 5 days and repeated every 6 weeks. The dose should be reduced if bone marrow toxicity is observed. **Polycythemia Vera:** For induction of remission, oral doses of 6 mg to 10 mg daily for 5 to 7 days have been used, then 2 mg to 4 mg daily until satisfactory disease control is achieved. For maintenance of therapy, 2 mg to 6 mg per week are given.

Storage: Under refrigeration.

Route of administration/infusion time: VO.

Reconstitution: NA.

Stability after reconstitution: NA.

Dilution: NA.

Stability after dilution: NA.

Recommendations: Because Alkeran is a potent myelosuppressive agent, it is essential that careful attention be paid to blood cell counts to avoid the possibility of excessive myelosuppression and the risk of irreversible medullary aplasia. Blood counts may continue to fall after treatment is stopped. Therefore, at the first sign of a sharp drop in WBC or platelet counts, treatment should be temporarily stopped. It should be used with caution in patients who have recently undergone radiotherapy or chemotherapy, in view of the increased toxicity to the bone marrow. Gastrointestinal effects, including nausea, vomiting, and diarrhea, are probably the most common signs of an acute oral overdose. The main toxic effect is bone marrow suppression, leading to leukopenia, thrombocytopenia, and anemia.

Main adverse reactions: Bone marrow suppression causing leukopenia, thrombocytopenia, and anemia; Nausea, vomiting, diarrhea, stomatitis (at high doses); Alopecia (at high doses). Gastrointestinal effects such as nausea and vomiting have been reported in more than 30% of patients being treated with conventional doses of melphalan. Temporary significant elevation of blood urea has been observed in the early stages of treatment with melphalan in patients with myeloma and renal damage; Alopecia (at conventional doses). Hemolytic anemia; urticaria, edema, skin rash and anaphylactic shock;

MERCAPTOPURINE

Trade Name/Presentation: Purinethol 50mg/tablet.

Therapeutic Class: Antineoplastic, Antimetabolite.

Indication: acute lymphoid leukemia.

Usual Dose: Children: Induction 2,5 - 5 mg/Kg/day or 60 - 75mg/m^2 / day. Maintenance: 1.5 - 2.5mg/m^2 /day. Adults: Induction 2.5 - 5.0mg/ g/day or 80 - 100mg/m^2 /day. Maintenance: 1.5 - 2.5mg/ kg/day.

Storage: TA.

Route of administration/infusion time: VO.

Reconstitution: NA.

Stability after reconstitution: NA.

Dilution: NA.

Stability after dilution: NA.

Recommendations: Take preferably on an empty stomach (1h before or 2h after meals). The main side effect of mercaptopurine treatment is bone marrow suppression, which causes leukopenia and thrombocytopenia. The incidence of hepatotoxicity varies considerably and can occur at any dose, but most frequently when the recommended daily dose of 2.5 mg/kg body weight or 75 mg/m2 body surface area is exceeded.

Main adverse reactions: Weakness, nausea and vomiting. Secondary leukemia and myelodysplasia. Medullary depression, leukopenia and thrombocytopenia. arthralgia, skin rash, drug fever. Facial edema. Anorexia. Nausea, vomiting, pancreatitis in patients with inflammatory bowel disease. Mouth ulceration, pancreatitis. Intestinal ulceration. Biliary cholestasis, hepatotoxicity. Hepatic necrosis

MESNA

Trade Name/Presentation: Mitexan: Ampoule in 100mg/mL concentration (4mL ampoule). Mesna: Ampoule in 100mg/mL concentration (4mL ampoule).

Therapeutic Category: Antidote.

Indication: Protection against hemorrhagic cystitis induced by the use of Ifosfamide and/or Cyclophosphamide.

Usual Dose: Adults and Children: 60% of the ifosfamide/cyclophosphamide dose divided into 3 administrations: the first dose (20%) is given IV at the same time as ifosfamide/cyclophosphamide; the 2nd dose (20%), 4h later, and the 3rd dose (20%), 8h after ifosfamide/cyclophosphamide administration. Other regimens can be used, such as continuous infusion of Mesna, employing a dose equivalent to that of Ifosfamide/Cyclophosphamide.

Storage: TA.

Route of administration/infusion time: Direct intravenous injection, 15-30 min infusion, or continuous infusion.

Simple equipment.

Reconstitution: NA.

Stability after reconstitution: NA.

Dilution: SF0, 9% or SG5% to a final concentration of 1-20mg/mL.

Stability after dilution: Until 25°: 24 Hs.

Recommendations: The protective effect of mesna is restricted to the urinary tract only. All other prophylactic or concomitant measures recommended for treatment with oxazafosforins are not affected and should therefore be maintained.

Main adverse reactions: Mesna rarely causes side effects if used correctly. Only when the individual dose of 60 mg/kg of body weight is exceeded can nausea, vomiting and diarrhea occur.

METOTREXATE

Trade Name/Presentation: Fauldmetro Injectable 50mg - 25mg/mL (2mL bottle).

Injectable 500mg - 25mg/mL Fauldmetro (20mL vial)

Methotrexate 2.5mg/tablet

Therapeutic Class: Antineoplastic, Antimetabolite.

Indication: acute lymphocytic leukemia; breast, lung, head and neck cancer; osteosarcoma; non-Hodgkin lymphoma; choriocarcinoma; osteosarcoma, autoimmune diseases and severe psoriasis, treatment of gestational choriocarcinoma, chorioadenoma destruens, and Mola Hydatiformis. Among others.

Usual Dose: Dose varies according to the chemotherapy protocol defined by the doctor. There is a great variability of doses and treatment schemes. Low conventional doses: 10 to 60mg/m^2, VO, IM, IV. Intermediate doses: 100 to 500mg/m^2, IV. High doses: 500mg up to 15g/m^2, IV. Intratecal: 10 to 15mg/m^2. Psoriasis: 10 to 25mg VO once a week, until adequate response achieved. Do not exceed 30mg/week. Rheumatoid arthritis: 7.5mg VO once a week. Do not exceed 20mg/week.

Storage: TA.

Route of administration/infusion time: Route of administration: VO, IV, IM, IT (intrathecal), IA (intra arterial), intraperitoneal and intravesical.

Simple equipment.

Reconstitution: Ready to use.

Stability after reconstitution: Under refrigeration: 24 Hs.

Dilution: SF0, 9% or SG 5%.

Stability after dilution: RT: 24Hs.

Recommendations: Intermediate and high doses require "rescue" with leucovorin. High doses of methotrexate should be accompanied by pre- and post-administration urine alkalinization as a preventive measure. Methotrexate can cause severe toxicity. Toxic effects may be related in frequency and severity to dose or periodicity of administration, but they have been observed at all dosages. Because these effects can occur at any time during therapy, it is necessary to carefully monitor patients taking methotrexate.

Main adverse reactions: Ulcerative stomatitis, leukopenia, nausea, and abdominal discomfort, as well as malaise, fatigue, fever and chills, dizziness, and decreased resistance to infection. Other adverse effects frequently reported are malaise, chills and fever, dizziness, and decreased resistance to infection. Gingivitis, pharyngitis, stomatitis, anorexia, nausea, vomiting, diarrhea, hematemesis, melena, gastrointestinal ulceration and bleeding, enteritis, and pancreatitis. Headache, drowsiness, blurred vision. Aphasia, hemiparesis, paresis and convulsions have also been reported after administration of Methotrexate. After small doses, some patients have reported transient cognitive dysfunction, mood alteration, or unusual cranial sensations. Conjunctivitis and visual changes of unknown etiology. Interstitial pneumonia and cases of chronic obstructive interstitial lung disease. Erythema, pruritus, urticaria, photosensitivity, pigmentary changes, alopecia, ecchymosis, telangiectasia, acne, furunculosis, erythema multiforme, Stevens Johnson syndrome. Renal failure, severe nephropathy, azotemia, cystitis, hematuria, impaired oogenesis or spermatogenesis, transient oligospermia, menstrual dysfunction, vaginal discharge, infertility, abortion, and fetal defects.

MITOMICINE

Trade Name/Presentation: Mitocin: Vial containing 5mg of lyophilized powder.

Therapeutic Category: Antineoplastic, Antibiotic.

Indication: Adenocarcinoma of stomach or pancreas, in combinations with other approved chemotherapeutic agents. Superficial transitional cell carcinoma of the urinary bladder.

Usual Dose: Intravenous: $20mg/m^2$, as a single dose, at intervals of 6-8 weeks. Intravesical: recommended 20mg-40mg at a concentration of 1mg/mL sterile water, 1 time/week for 8 weeks.

Storage: TA.

Route of administration/infusion time: IV bolus (3 to 4 minutes) or under continuous infusion (30 minutes). Intra-arterial. Intraperitoneal. Intrapleural. Intravesical.

Photoresist Equipo.

Reconstitution: Reconstitute each vial with 10mL of ABD, resulting in a concentration of 0.5mg/mL.

Stability after reconstitution: Under refrigeration: 48 Hs.

Dilution: 50 to 250 mL of 0.9% SF.

Stability after dilution: 12 hours T. A. (SF 0.9%) and 3 hours (SG 5%).

Recommendations: Avoid SG 5% as stability is lower (3 Hs). In intravesical administration use Nacl 0.9% (concentration 1 mg;mL).

Main adverse reactions: Fever; nausea; diarrhea; loss of appetite; inflammation in the mouth; decreased platelets in the blood; decreased leukocytes in the blood; pain at the injection site; reversible hair loss.

MITOXANTRONE

Trade Name/Presentation: Evomixan vial in the concentration 20mg - 2mg/mL (10mL vial).
Therapeutic Class: Antineoplastic, Antibiotic (anthracenedione).
Indication: Leukemias, breast carcinoma, including locally advanced and metastatic disease.
Usual Dose: The recommended starting dose for single agent use is 14 mg/m2 body surface area, given as a single intravenous dose, which may be repeated at 21-day intervals. A lower starting dose (12 mg/m2 or less) is recommended in patients with inadequate spinal cord reserves due to previous therapy or poor general condition. When used in combination chemotherapy with another myelosuppressive agent, the starting dose of mitoxantrone should be reduced 2 to 4 mg/m2 below the doses recommended for use as a single agent.
Storage: Under refrigeration.
Route of administration/infusion time: Intrapleural. Intravesical. IV bolus or IV continuous infusion 15 to 30 minutes.
Single Equipo.
Reconstitution: Ready to use.
Stability after reconstitution: NA.
Dilution: 100 mL of 0.9% SF or 5% SG.
Stability after dilution: RT: 48 Hs.
Recommendation: A hemopoietic, gastrointestinal, hepatic or renal toxicity may be observed depending on the dose administered and the physical condition of the patient.
Main adverse reactions: A certain degree of leukopenia should be expected after the recommended doses. Thrombocytopenia is also reversible. Nausea and vomiting. anorexia, diarrhea, gastrointestinal bleeding and stomatitis/mucositis. Hypotension, urticaria and exanthema have occasionally been reported.

ONCO BCG

Trade Name/Presentation: Imuno BCG: Vial containing 40 MG lyophilized GCG.

Therapeutic Category: Immunobiologicals.

Indication: Treatment of primary/recurrent flat urothelial carcinoma of the bladder "in situ". Adjuvant treatment after resection of primary or recurrent TA T1 grade 1, 2 or 3 superficial urothelial carcinoma of the bladder.

Usual Dose: 80 MG= 2 ampoules of 1 mL each re-suspended in 50 ml of sterile physiological solution, without preservative.

Storage: Under refrigeration.

Route of administration/infusion time: Intravesical route. Treatment time may vary from 8 to 12 weeks. Instill 50 ml of IMUNO BCG suspension aseptically, via urethral tube, slowly into the empty bladder, taking care never to force the flow. At the end of the instillation, the urethral tube is removed, and the patient is instructed to retain the suspension in the bladder for 2 hours. To ensure that the medication is most effective, try to rest for 15 minutes in each position (face down, back, left side, right side). Restriction of fluid intake 3-6 hours before instillation may be recommended for patients with limited bladder capacity. Since IMUNO BCG is not a biohazard material, the suspension can be purged normally and no special precautions are necessary.

Reconstitution: Resuspend 2 vials of IMUNO BCG in 50 ml of physiological solution (NaCl 0.9%) without preservative, in a sterile area using aseptic technique during the whole procedure. Proceed with reconstitution of each vial of IMUNO BCG as follows:

1 - Lightly tap the ampoule so that the lithophil is deposited at the bottom of the ampoule; 2 - Clean the opening site of the ampoule with a gauze or cotton moistened in alcohol; 3 - Check if the opening site is dry. Wrap the ampoule with the plastic bag that comes with it, breaking it at the rupture point; 4 - Remove the plastic bag slowly, in order to allow the air to penetrate the ampoule gradually.

Slowly inject through the wall of the ampoule 2 drops of diluent, with a sterile disposable syringe, in order to moisten the lymophil. Then, add a little more of the diluent, slowly shaking until a homogeneous suspension is obtained. Finally, slowly inject the rest of the diluent (2-3 ml.). AVOID VIGOROUS AGITATION.

Stability after reconstitution: After reconstitution of IMUNO BCG, store at 2 to 8°C and do not expose to light. The suspension should be used as soon as possible (maximum time for use is 4 h).

Dilution: Transfer the contents of the 2 vials into a sterile, disposable 50 ml syringe. Add a volume of sterile physiological solution, up to the total volume of 50 ml. The suspension should be homogeneous and slightly opaque.

Stability after dilution: Immediate use.

Recommendations: It should not be administered intravenously, subcutaneously or intramuscularly due to the risks of occurrence of serious adverse events. Aseptic insertion of the tube should be performed without trauma to avoid damage to the bladder surface and urothelium. Immunotherapy with BCG should be discontinued until a systemic infection has been excluded. Treatment with IMUNO BCG should be discontinued at least within 7-14 days after urothelium trauma due to bladder biopsy, transurethral resection, traumatic catheterization, or bladder injury, as treatment with BCG after the above invasive procedures may result in systemic BCG infection. For patients at risk for HIV infection, HIV testing is recommended before starting treatment with IMUNO BCG. USE IN THE Elderly, CHILDREN AND OTHER RISK GROUPS Use in pregnant and lactating women is not recommended because there are no data on the effect on the fetus or excretion in human milk. IMUNO BCG cannot be administered to patients with immune deficiency

Main Adverse Reactions: Mild to moderate transient reactions: The reactions described below are generally mild to moderate, usually lasting no longer than 2 days, and are believed to be the result of a positive immune response to BCG. Local side effects such as dysuria, increased urinary frequency, cystitis, and hematuria are common. Systemic reactions such as fever and chills can occur in a significant number of cases, and malaise and myalgia can also occur. Antipyretics, fluids, and/or analgesics can be used to treat these symptoms. Moderate side effects can also be treated prophylactically with 300 mg isoniazid for 3 days. Rare and uncommon side effects: Related complications are rarely seen, occurring most often after 3 or more instillations, or related to the maintenance regimen. Fever above 39°C, which does not disappear after 24-48 hours after the patient is given fluids and antipyretics, and/or a period with malaise and fever, during which symptoms increase, may indicate a systemic infection. Immunotherapy with BCG should be discontinued until a systemic infection has been ruled out. Immunotherapy can be restarted with caution if necessary. Allergic reactions such as arthralgia, myalgia or rash occur in very few patients. Macroscopic hematuria, bladder contracture or temporary urethral obstructions are also rare complications. Localized BCG infections such as prostatitis or epididymo-orchitis or systemic reactions (including hepatitis or pneumonia) are extremely rare, but require immediate discontinuation of immunotherapy and consultation with an infectious disease specialist for treatment with antituberculosis therapy. Systemic BCG infection can be a life-threatening complication. Immediate institution of triple anti-tuberculosis treatment together with 100 mg prednisone per day is recommended.

OXALIPLATIN

Trade Name/Presentation: Oxalibbs vial containing 50 and 100 MG.

Therapeutic Class: Antineoplastic, Alkylating agent.

Indication: metastatic colorectal cancer in association or not with fluoropyrimidines.

Usual Dose: 130mg/m2, either in monotherapy or in association with other chemotherapy drugs. The interval varies according to the chemotherapy protocol defined by the doctor.

Storage: TA.

Route of administration/infusion time: Administer in a venous infusion every 2-6 hours.

Simple equipment.

Reconstitution: Reconstitute 50mg with 20mL of ABD, and 100mg with 40mL of ABD.

Stability after reconstitution: Under refrigeration: 48h .

Dilution: 250 to 500mL of SGI 5%.

Stability after dilution: RT: 24 Hs.

Recommendations: Perform the infusion of oxaliplatin before fluorouracil. Medication incompatible with SF 0.9%.

Main Adverse Reactions: Anemia, neutropenia, thrombocytopenia. Acute neurosensory symptoms. Dysesthesia/paresthesia of extremities and peripheral neuropathy. Dysgeusia. Coughing. Acute interstitial lung disease, pulmonary fibrosis Nausea, vomiting, diarrhea Dehydration, hypokalemia, metabolic acidosis, paralytic ileus, intestinal obstruction, and renal disorders may be associated with severe diarrhea/vomiting, particularly when it is combined with 5-fluorouracil. Stomatitis, mucositis Abdominal pain Gastrointestinal bleeding Alopecia Back pain In the case of such an adverse reaction, hemolysis, which has rarely been reported, should be investigated Arthralgia. Epistaxis Anorexia Deep vein thrombosis

Thromboembolic events hypertension fatigue Fever, stiffness (tremors), due to infection (with or without febrile neutropenia) or possibly from the immune mechanism Asthenia. Injection site reactions. Injection site reactions including local pain, redness, swelling and thrombosis have been reported. Allergic reactions such as: skin rash (particularly urticaria), conjunctivitis, rhinitis. Anaphylactic reactions including bronchospasm, chest pain sensation, angioedema, hypotension, anaphylactic shock. Hemolytic uremic syndrome. Seizure.

PACLITAXEL

Trade Name/Presentation: Evotaxel: Vial containing 300 MG/50 mL.

Ontax: Ampoule vial containing 150, 100 and 30 MG.

Therapeutic Class: Antineoplastic, Taxane (antimicrobial agent).

Indication: Metastatic ovarian carcinoma, breast cancer, head and neck cancer, and lung cancer.

Usual Dose: 80mg/m2 to 225mg/m2 every 3 weeks. The dose varies according to the chemotherapy protocol defined by the doctor.

Storage: TA.

Route of administration/infusion time: doses between 135mg/m2 to 175mg/m2 are commonly infused in 3h. Doses < than 90mg/m2 are usually infused in 1h.

Equipo exempt of PVC.

Reconstitution: NA.

Stability after reconstitution: 28 days under refrigeration (Evotaxel). 24 Hs RT (Ontax).

Dilution: Dilute in SS, SG, SGF, or Ringer's solution to a final concentration of 0.3-1.2 mg/mL.

Stability after dilution: RT: 24 Hs (Evotaxel). RT: 27 Hs (Ontax). (Do not refrigerate diluted solutions).

Recommendation: Contact of the undiluted concentrate with PVC (polyvinyl chloride) plastic materials or devices used in the preparation of infusion solutions is not recommended. Patients should be treated with corticosteroids, antihistamines and H2 antagonists prior to the administration of paclitaxel. In the institution usually used in the preparation of the paclitaxel infusion is ondasentrona, dexamethasone 20 mg, diphenhydramine 50 mg and ranitidine 50mg or cimetidine 300mg.

Main adverse reactions: Dyspnea requiring bronchodilators, hypotension requiring treatment, angioedema or generalized urticaria. Bone marrow depression (mainly neutropenia). Hypotension, hypertension and bradycardia. Peripheral neuropathy.

PAMIDRONATE

Trade Name/Presentation: Disodium Pamidronate/Aredia: Ampoule containing 30mg of lyophilized powder.

Therapeutic Class: Bone resorption inhibitor.

Indication: treatment of conditions associated with increased osteoclastic activity: bone metastases, hypercalcemia, and Paget's disease.

Usual Dose: Bone metastases: recommended dose 90 mg every 4 to 3 weeks. The total dose depends on the patient's serum calcium levels.

Storage: TA.

Route of administration/Infusion time: Do not exceed a concentration of 90mg in 250mL. Can be infused in 90 min or up to 3 Hs.

Simple equipment.

Reconstitution: Reconstitute with 10mL of sterile water for injection (included with the product).

Stability after reconstitution: Under refrigeration: 24 Hs.

Dilution: SF0.9% and SG5%.

Stability after dilution: RT: 24hs.

Recommendations: Do not administer in bolus and do not exceed 1mg/min.

Main Adverse Reactions: These are usually mild and transient. The most common adverse reactions are: flu-like symptoms with mild fever; headache; nausea; vomiting; infusion site reactions (pain, redness, swelling, induration).

PEMETREXEDE

Trade Name/Presentation: Alimta vial containing lyophilized powder in concentrations of 100 and 500mg.

Therapeutic Class: Antineoplastic agent, antifolate.

Indication: Pleural mesothelioma.

Usual Dose: 500mg/m2 every 28 days.

Combined use with cisplatin

The recommended dose of ALIMTA is 500 mg/m2, administered by intravenous infusion over 10 minutes on the first day of each 21-day cycle. The recommended dose of cisplatin is 75 mg/m2 by intravenous infusion over 2 hours, starting approximately 30 minutes after the end of ALIMTA administration on the first day of each 21-day cycle.

Single agent

The recommended dose of ALIMTA is 500 mg/m2, administered by intravenous infusion over 10 minutes, on the first day of each 21-day cycle. Treatment with ALIMTA should be continued until progression of the underlying disease.

Storage: TA.

Route of administration/infusion time: Infusion: IV 10 minutes.

Reconstitution: 20mL SF0.9% (concentration: 25mg/mL).

Stability after reconstitution: RT: 24 Hs.

Dilution: 100mL SF0.9%.

Stability after dilution: RT: 24 Hs.

Recommendation: Reconstitution and subsequent dilution prior to intravenous infusion is only recommended with 0.9% injectable sodium chloride (without preservative). ALIMTA is physically incompatible with calcium-containing diluents, including Ringer Lactate and Ringer, which should therefore not be used. It may suppress bone marrow function, and neutropenia, thrombocytopenia, and anemia (or pancytopenia) may occur; myelosuppression is usually the dose-limiting toxicity.

Main Adverse Reactions: Blood and Lymphatic System Changes. Ocular Changes (Conjunctivitis). Gastrointestinal Changes. Fatigue. Dehydration. Sensory Neuropathy. Taste Disorder. Creatinine elevation. Cutaneous eruption. Alopecia.

RITUXIMABE

Trade Name/Presentation: Mabthera Injectable 100mg - 10mg/mL (10mL vial)

Mabthera Injectable 500mg - 10mg/mL (50mL vial)

Therapeutic Class: Antineoplastic, Monoclonal antibody.

Indication: B-cell, low-grade or follicular, CD20-positive, relapsed or refractory to chemotherapy and diffuse large-cell, intermediate or high-grade, CD20-positive, non-Hodgkin's lymphomas associated with the CHOP or EPOCH protocol.

Usual Dose: 375mg/m2/week for 4 weeks.

Storage: Under refrigeration.

Administration route/infusion time: the first infusion should start slowly and gradually be accelerated to prevent and control adverse reactions. It is recommended to start at a rate of 50 mg/h, increase by 50 mg/h every 30 minutes up to a maximum of 400 mg/h. Subsequent infusions can be started at a rate of 100 mg/h, with increments of 100 mg/h every 30 minutes up to a maximum of 400 mg/h.

Reconstitution: Ready to use.

Stability after reconstitution: Immediate use.

Dilution: 0.9% SF or 5% SG at a concentration of 1-4 mg/mL.

Stability after dilution: 12h RT or 24 SR.

Recommendations: should be preceded by pre-medication, 30-60min before, consisting of an analgesic (e.g. paracetamol) and an antihistamine drug (e.g. diphenhydramine).

Main Adverse Reactions: Bacterial infections, viral infections. Sepsis, pneumonia, febrile infection, shingles, respiratory tract infections, fungal infections, infections of unknown etiology. Neutropenia, leukopenia. Anemia, thrombocytopenia. Coagulation disorders, transient aplastic anemia, hemolytic anemia, lymphadenopathy. Angioedema. Hypersensitivity. Hyperglycemia, weight loss, peripheral edema, facial edema, increased LDH, hypocalcemia. Depression, nervousness. Paresthesia, hypoesthesia, agitation, insomnia, vasodilation, dizziness, anxiety. Dysgeusia. Paresthesia, hypoesthesia, agitation, insomnia, vasodilation, dizziness, anxiety. Tearing disorder, conjunctivitis. Tinnitus, otalgia. Myocardial infarction, arrhythmia, atrial fibrillation, tachycardia, cardiac disorder Left ventricular failure, supraventricular tachycardia, ventricular tachycardia, angina, myocardial ischemia, bradycardia Hypertension, orthostatic hypotension, hypotension. Bronchospasm, respiratory illness, chest pain, dyspnea, cough, rhinitis. Asthma, bronchiolitis obliterans, lung disorder, hypoxia Nausea. Vomiting, diarrhea, abdominal pain, dysphagia, stomatitis, dyspepsia, constipation, anorexia, throat irritation. Enlargement of the abdomen. Pruritus, *rash*. Urticaria, alopecia, sweating, night sweats. Hypertonia, myalgia, arthralgia, back pain, neck pain, aches, Fever, chills, asthenia, headache, Tumor pain, flushing, malaise, cold, Pain at the infusion site, Reduced IgG levels.

<h1 align="center">TAMOXYFEN</h1>

Trade Name/Presentation: Tamoxifen: 10 mg tablet.

Therapeutic Category: Antineoplastic, Hormone.

Indication: treatment of breast cancer.

Usual Dose: Adults and elderly: 20mg/day in a single dose. After 1 or 2 months, if there is no satisfactory response, the dose may be increased to 20mg, twice a day.

Storage: TA.

Route of administration/infusion time: VO.

Reconstitution: NA.

Stability after reconstitution: NA.

Dilution: NA.

Stability after dilution: NA.

Recommendations: This medicine should be taken with water, preferably at the same time each day. It should not be broken or chewed. Seek medical attention immediately if: Difficulty breathing with or without swelling of the face, lips, tongue and/or throat. Swelling of the face, lips, tongue, and/or throat causing difficulty swallowing. Swelling in the hands, feet, or ankles. Having redness of the skin.

Major Adverse Reactions: Heat waves. Stroke, clogging of deep veins in the leg and lung, vaginal bleeding, vaginal discharge, itching in the vagina, changes in the uterine wall (including thickening and polyps), gastrointestinal intolerance (stomach upsets, including nausea and vomiting), hair loss, skin rashes (rashes on the skin or itching or peeling of the skin), headache, dizziness, redness of the tumor area, fluid retention (possibly seen as swollen ankles), and cramps. Cataracts, retinopathy, uterine fibroids (which can also be seen as pelvic discomfort or vaginal bleeding), endometrial cancer (inner lining of the uterine wall), allergic reactions, abnormal decrease in the number of platelets in the blood, decrease in the number of WBCs in the blood, abnormal decrease in the number of neutrophils in the blood, anemia, changes in liver enzyme rates, and elevation of triglycerides. Corneal changes, optic nerve disease and inflammation, uterine sarcoma (malignant tumors), endometriosis, ovarian cysts, pancreatitis (inflammation of the pancreas), fatty liver, decreased bile flow, hepatitis, and elevated calcium in the blood. Inflammation of the lungs, which can have symptoms such as pneumonia, shortness of breath, and coughing; severe skin changes (such as redness, blisters, and peeling).

TEMOZOLAMIDE

Trade name/ Presentation: Temodal 5mg , 20mg, 100mg, 250mg capsule.

Therapeutic Class: Antineoplastic, alkylating agent.

Indication: Treatment of patients with brain tumors (malignant glioma, anaplastic astrocytoma, glioblastoma multiforme) and mestatic melanoma.

Usual Dose: 75mg - 200mg/m2/day, according to therapeutic indication.

Storage: TA.

Route of administration/infusion time: VO.

Reconstitution: NA.

Stability after reconstitution: NA.

Dilution: NA.

Stability after dilution: NA.

Recommendations: Capsules can be taken independently of food, however, administration one hour before a meal may assist in reducing nausea. Capsules should be taken whole, always at the same time. Administer with caution in patients with severe hepatic and renal impairment.

Main Adverse Reactions: Oral candidiasis, infection. Oral candidiasis, herpes simplex, infection, pharyngitis, infected sores, Herpes simplex or shingles, cold-like symptoms. Leukopenia, lymphopenia, neutropenia, thrombocytopenia Anemia, febrile neutropenia, leukopenia, thrombocytopenia Anemia, febrile neutropenia Lymphopenia, petechiae. Cushing's syndrome. Anorexia. Hyperglycemia, weight loss Hypokalemia, increased alkaline phosphatase, weight gain. Weight loss Hyperglycemia, weight gain Anxiety, emotional lability, insomnia Agitation, apathy, behavioral changes, depression, hallucination Anxiety, depression, emotional lability, insomnia Hallucination, amnesia. Headache. Convulsion Dizziness, aphasia, altered balance, difficulty concentrating, confusion, dysphagia, hemiparesis, difficulty memorizing, neurological disorders, neuropathy, peripheral neuropathy, paresthesia, drowsiness, altered speech, tremors Ataxia, impaired cognition, dysphagia, extrapyramidal disorders, abnormal gait, hemiparesis, hyperesthesia, hypoesthesia, neurological disorders, peripheral neuropathy, epilepsy. Sensory disorder. Blurred vision. Eye pain, hemianopia, visual disorder, reduction in visual acuity, visual field defect. Difficulty hearing Tinnitus. Otalgia, hyperacusis, tinnitus, otitis media Deafness, otalgia, vertigo Palpitation. Lower limb edema, hemorrhage, deep vein thrombosis Hypertension, cerebral hemorrhage. Edema, peripheral edema, pulmonary embolism. Pneumonia, upper respiratory tract infection, nasal congestion, sinusitis, bronchitis, constipation, nausea, vomiting Abdominal pain, diarrhea, dyspepsia, dysphagia, stomatitis Diarrhea, dyspepsia, dysphagia, dry mouth, stomatitis Abdominal distention,

fecal incontinence, gastrointestinal disorder, gastroenteritis, hemorrhoids. Alopecia, exanthema. Dry skin, pruritus. Dermatitis, dry skin, erythema, pruritus. Photosensitivity reaction, abnormal pigmentation, skin exfoliation. Erythema, abnormal pigmentation, increased sweating. Arthralgia, musculoskeletal pain, myalgia, muscle weakness Muscle weakness. Back pain, musculoskeletal pain, myalgia, myopathy Back pain, myopathy Frequent urination, urinary incontinence Urinary incontinence Dysuria. Impotence Fatigue. Fever, pain, allergic reaction, radiotherapy injury, face edema, taste perversion Erythema, flushing, worsening asthenia, chills, discoloration of tongue, parosmia, thirst. Worsening asthenia, pain, chills, dental change, facial edema, taste perversion. Increased TGPs. Increased Gamma- GT, increased liver enzymes, increased TGOs

TIOGUANINE

Trade Name/Presentation: Lanvis 40mg/tablet.

Therapeutic Class: Antineoplastic, Antimetabolite.

Indication: Myeloblastic leukemia and acute lymphoblastic leukemia.

Usual Dose: For adults and children, the usual dose is 2.0-2.5g/ kg/day, but the dose and duration of administration depend on the nature and dose of other cytotoxic agents administered in conjunction with Lanvis.

Storage: TA.

Route of administration/infusion time: NA.

Reconstitution: NA.

Stability after reconstitution: NA.

Dilution: NA.

Stability after dilution: NA.

Recommendations: Take with a little water and well in advance of meals.

Main adverse reactions: Bone marrow suppression. Gastrointestinal stomatitis and intolerance. Intestinal necrosis and perforations. Liver toxicity associated with endothelial vascular damage when thioguanine is used in maintenance or long-term continued therapy, which is not recommended. Liver toxicity usually appears as a clinical syndrome of hepatic veno-occlusive disease (hyperbilirubinemia, painful hepatomegaly, weight gain due to fluid retention, and ascites) or with signs of portal hypertension (splenomegaly, thrombocytopenia, and esophageal varices). Elevation of liver transaminases, alkaline phosphatase and gamma-glutamyltransferase, and jaundice may also occur. Histopathologic features associated with this toxicity include hepatoportal sclerosis, regenerative nodular hyperplasia, hapatic pelliosis, and periportal fibrosis. Hepatic toxicity during a therapeutic cycle is of short duration, appearing as a veno-occlusive disease. Reversal of the symptoms and signs of this hepatic toxicity has been reported with discontinuation of therapy, whether of short or long duration. Centrilobular hepatic necrosis has been reported in some cases including patients receiving combination chemotherapy, oral contraceptives, high doses of thioguanine, and alcohol.

TOPOTECANE

Trade Name/Presentation: Hycantim: vial containing 4 mg lyophilized powder.

Therapeutic Class: Antineoplastic, Topoisomerase I inhibitor.

Indication: metastatic ovarian carcinoma, myelodysplastic syndromes, and brain tumors.

Usual Dose: 1.5mg/m2/day, IV, for 5 consecutive days, starting on day 1 of a 21-day cycle. A minimum of 4 cycles is recommended. 1.3-1.6mg/m2/day, IV, in a 30 min, 2h or 24h infusion, every 3-4 weeks. 1.5 to 1.75mg/m2/day, IV, in 24h infusion, weekly. 0.65 to 2.0mg/m2/day, IV, in 72-, 96-, or 120-h continuous infusion, every 3-4 weeks.

Storage: TA.

Administration route/infusion time: IV: 30 min or continuous infusion as per protocol.

Photoresist Equipo.

Reconstitution: each vial contains 4 mL of ABD.

Stability after reconstitution: Immediate use.

Dilution: Dilution: SF0.9% or SG5%, concentration: 0.02 to 0.5 mg/ mL.

Stability after dilution: 24 Hs Under refrigeration.

Recommendations: Inadvertent blood extravasation has been associated with only mild local reactions such as erythema and petechiae. Caution should be exercised when driving and operating machinery if fatigue and asthenia persist.

Main adverse reactions: Neutropenia. Leukopenia. Thrombocytopenia. Anemia. Sepsis or fever/infection with grade 4 neutropenia. Platelet transfusions. Red blood cell transfusions Nausea (which may be severe) Vomiting (may be severe) Diarrhea (can be severe)

Constipation abdominal pain Stomatitis. Anorexia (can be serious) Fatigue fever Pain. Asthenia. Alopecia. rash Dyspnea cough headache

TRASTUZUMAB

Trade Name/Presentation: Herceptin: vial containing440mgn of lyophilized powder.

Therapeutic Class: Antineoplastic, Monoclonal antibody.

Indication: Metastatic breast cancer presenting tumors with HER2 overexpression and other metastatic tumors.

Usual Dose: 1 - Initial loading dose: 8mg/kg over 90 minutes. Subsequent doses: 6mg/kg in 30-90 minutes (30min if well tolerated in previous infusions). 2 - Start dose: 4mg/kg, in 90min infusion, subsequent doses: 2mg/kg/week, in 30min infusion (if well tolerated in previous infusions).

Storage: Under refrigeration.

Route of administration/infusion time: IV: 30 - 90 Minutes.

Simple equipment.

Reconstitution: Reconstitute with the accompanying diluent or ABD. The resulting solution is 21mg/mL.

Stability after reconstitution: 28 days, under refrigeration if reconstituted with proper diluent and 24 Hs with ABD.

Dilution: Further dilution in 250 mL of 0.9% SF. Do not use SG 5%. Introduce the drug slowly and to mix the solution, invert the vial slowly, avoiding the formation of foam.

Stability after dilution: 24 Hs under refrigeration or RT.

Recommendations: Do not administer as a rapid intravenous injection or bolus. Conditions that require caution during administration: possibility of difficulty in breathing, low blood pressure, wheezing, bronchial spasm and tachycardia, among other symptoms.

Main adverse reactions: dyspnea, hypotension, wheezing, bronchospasm, tachycardia, reduced oxygen saturation, and respiratory failure. interstitial lung disease, including lung infiltrates, acute respiratory distress syndrome, pneumonia, pneumonitis, pleural effusion, shortness of breath, acute pulmonary edema, and respiratory failure. Heart failure. Infusion-related symptoms such as fever and chills, usually after the first infusion. Abdominal pain, asthenia, chest pain, chills, fever, headache, pain, diarrhea, nausea, vomiting, arthralgia, myalgia, dorsalgia, flu-like syndrome, infection, cervicalgia, malaise, hypersensitivity reactions, vasodilation, supraventricular tachyarrhythmia, hypotension, heart failure, cardiomyopathy, palpitation, anorexia, constipation, dyspepsia, leukopenia, peripheral edema, edema, bone pain, anxiety, depression, dizziness, insomnia, paresthesia, somnolence, hypertonia, peripheral neuropathy, asthma, cough exacerbation, dyspnea, epistaxis, lung disorders, pleural effusion, pharyngitis, rhinitis, sinusitis, urinary tract infection, pruritus, sweating, ungual alterations, dry skin, alopecia, acne, maculopapular exanthema.

VIMBLASTIN

Trade Name/Presentation: Faulblastine 1mg/mL Injectable - 10mL vial.

Therapeutic Class: Antineoplastic, Vinca alkaloid.

Indication: Hodgkin's disease, Lymphocytic lymphoma, advanced testicular carcinoma and Kaposi's sarcoma.

Usual Dose: Adults: 3.7mg/m2 with gradual weekly increase up to $11.1mg/m^2$. Maximum dose: $18.5mg/m^2$. Children: $2.5mg/m^2$ with weekly increments up to $7.5mg/m^2$. Maximum dose: $12.5mg/m^2$. Doses vary according to the chemotherapy protocol defined by the physician.

Storage: Under refrigeration.

Route of administration/infusion time: IV: administer the drug in short infusions (maximum 30min). For peripheral access: infuse parallel 250mL SF.

Simple equipment.

Reconstitution: Ready to use.

Stability after reconstitution: Immediate use.

Dilution: SF in a maximum volume of 100 mL.

Stability after dilution: Immediate use.

Recommendation: Due to the increased possibility of thrombosis, it is inadvisable to inject a vimblastine sulfate solution into an extremity in which circulation is impaired or potentially impaired by conditions such as compression, neoplasm invasion, phlebitis, or varicosity. INTRATHECAL ADMINISTRATION IS FATAL. FOR INTRAVENOUS USE ONLY.

Main adverse reactions: Leukopenia, anemia, thrombocytopenia (myelosuppression). Cellulitis and phlebitis, caused by extravasation during intravenous injection. If the amount of extravasation is large, local necrosis may occur. Alopecia, often not total. Constipation, anorexia, nausea and vomiting (easily controlled by antiemetic agents), abdominal pain, paralytic ileus, vesicles in the mouth, pharyngitis, diarrhea, hemorrhagic enterocolitis, bleeding from an existing peptic ulcer, and rectal bleeding. Tingling of the fingers (paresthesia), loss of deep tendon reflexes, peripheral neuritis, mental depression, headache, and convulsions. Hypertension. Acute dyspnea and severe bronchospasm Malaise, bone pain, weakness, tumor site pain, dizziness, jaw pain, skin vesiculation, hypertension, hyperuricemia, uric nephropathy, syndrome attributed to inappropriate secretion of antidiuretic hormone (occurred with higher than recommended doses) and Raynaud's phenomenon (in patients treated with vimblastine sulfate combined with bleomycin and cisplatin for testicular cancer).

VINCRISTINA

Trade Name/Presentation: Fauldvincri: vial in a 1mg/1mL concentration.

Tecnocris: vial in a 1mg/1mL concentration.

Therapeutic Class: Antineoplastic, Vinca alkaloid.

Indication: acute leukemia, Hodgkin's disease, malignant non-Hodgkin's lymphoma, rhabdomyosarcoma, neuroblastoma, Wilms' tumor, carcinoma, and melanoma, among others.

Usual Dose: Adults: $1.4mg/m^2$ weekly. Children: Weight > 10kg: 1.5 to $2.0mg/m^2$; Weight < 10kg or SC < $1m^2$: 0.05mg/kg weekly. Continuous infusion: 0.4mg/day, for 4 days (VAD protocol). It is recommended not to exceed a dose of 2.0mg per application.

Storage: Under refrigeration.

Route of administration/infusion time: Administration: Exclusively for intravenous use in push or under infusion. Peripheral access: Infuse parallel 250mL SF.

Simple equipment.

Reconstitution: Ready to use.

Stability after reconstitution: Tecnocris (Under refrigeration: 48 Hs). Faudvincri (Under refrigeration: 24 Hs).

Dilution: Further dilution, with 0.9% SF or 5% SG.

Stability after dilution: 4 days AT or under refrigeration.

Recommendations: should be administered exclusively intravenously, not intramuscularly, subcutaneously or intrathecally. Intrathecal administration can be fatal.

Main Adverse Reactions: Alopecia. Anaphylaxis, skin rash and edema. constipation, abdominal cramps, weight loss, nausea, vomiting, oral ulcerations, diarrhea, paralytic ileus, intestinal necrosis and/or perforation and anorexia. Polyuria, dysuria, and urinary retention due to bladder atony. Abdominal pain or colic, hypertension and hypotension.

VINORELBINA

Trade Name/Presentation: Evotabine: vial containing 50 mg/5 mL;

Navelbine: vial containing 50 mg/5 mL;

Therapeutic Class: Antineoplastic, Vinca alkaloid.

Indication: Non-small cell lung carcinoma and breast cancer.

Usual Dose: 25-30mg/m^2 /week, IV, as stand alone drug. 25- 30mg/m^2 /, IV, in combination with cisplatin 120mg/m^2 , on days 1 and 29, every six weeks.

Storage: TA.

Route of administration/infusion time: IV: 6-10min. Peripheral access: Infuse parallel 250mL SF.

Photoresist Equipo.

Reconstitution: Ready to use.

Stability after reconstitution: Under refrigeration or RT: 24 Hs.

Dilution: 0.9% SF or 5% SG in 1.5-3mg/mL concentration for syringe use and 0.5- 2mg/mL for saline solution application.

Stability after dilution: Evotabine: 24h TA. Navelbine: 24h under refrigeration.

Recommendations: May have additive bone marrow depressant effects with: other bone marrow depressants. May cause acute pulmonary reactions with: mitomycin May increase the risk of adverse reactions from: live virus vaccines.

Main adverse reactions: Weakness, fatigue, nerve problems. Lack of appetite, constipation, diarrhea, nausea, inflammation in mouth, vomiting. Decreased white blood cells in the blood, anemia Hair loss, pain or reaction at the injection site.

CARE MANAGEMENT

Order of Infusion of Chemotherapy

Infusion order	Medication
1st EV 60 minutes before 5FU	1° Folinic acid
2°	2ND 5FU

Order of infusion	Medication
1°	Irinotecan
2°	Folinic acid
3°	5FU

Infusion order	Medication
1°	Irinotecan
2°	Oxaliplatin

Infusion order	Medication
R-CHOP	
1°	Rituximab
2°	Doxorubicin
3°	Cyclophosphamide
4°	Vincristine
Prednisone 40mg/day VO days 1 to 5	

Infusion order	Medication
1°	Gencitabine
2°	Vinorelbine

Infusion order	Medication
1°	Docetaxel
2°	Gencitabine

Infusion order	Medication
1°	Paclitaxel
2°	Gencitabine

Infusion order	Medication
1°	Methotrexate
2°	5FU

Infusion order	Medication
MVAC	
1°	Metotexate
2°	Vimblastine
3°	Doxorubicin
4°	Cisplatin

Infusion order	Medication
ABVD	
1°	Adriamycin
2°	Bleomycin
3°	Vimblastine
4°	Dacarbazine

Infusion order	Medication
CMF	
1°	Cyclophosphamide
2°	Metrotexate
3°	Fluorouracil

Infusion order	Medication
1°	Adriamycin
2°	Fluorouracil
3°	Cyclophosphamide

Infusion order	Medication
1°	Methotrexate
2°	5FU

Infusion order	Medication
1°	Folinic acid
2°	5FU bolus
3°	Oxaliplatin
4°	5FU continuous inf.

Infusion order	Medication
1°	5FU
2°	Cisplatin

Infusion order	Medication
1°	Etoposide
2°	Carbo or cisplatin

Infusion order	Medication
TIP	
1°	Ifosfamide
2°	Mesna H0 (30' before IFO, H3 and H6)
3°	Cisplatin
4°	Taxol

Infusion order	Medication
1°	Docetaxel
2°	Ifosfamide

Infusion order	Medication
1°	Doxorubicin
2°	Cyclophosphamide
3°	Paclitaxel

Infusion order	Medication
CHOP	
1°	Doxorubicin
2°	Cyclophosphamide
3°	Vincristine
Prednisone 40mg/day VO days 1 to 5	

Infusion order	Medication
COP	
1°	Cyclophosphamide
2°	Vincristine
Prednisone 40mg/day VO days 1 to 5	

Infusion order	Medication
VeIP	
1°	Ifosfamide
2°	Mesna H0 (30' before IFO, H3 and H6)
3°	Vimblastine
4°	Cyclophosphamide

Infusion order	Medication
ELF	
1°	Vepesid
2°	Fluoruracil
3°	Leucovorin

Infusion order	Medication
VIP	
1°	Ifosfamide
2°	Mesna H0 (30' before IFO, H3 and H6)
3°	Etoposide
4°	Cisplatin

Infusion order	Medication
FAC	
1°	Doxorubicin
2°	Fluoruracil
3°	Cyclophosphamide

Infusion order	Medication
IFL	
1°	Irinotecan
2°	Fluoruracil
3°	Leucovorin

Infusion order	Medication
PEB	
1°	Etoposide
2°	Cisplatin
3°	Bleomycin

Infusion order	Medication
FLOX	
1°	Oxaliplatin
2°	Leucovorin Y w/ OXA
3°	Fluoruracil

Infusion order	Medication
CVD	
1°	Cisplatin
2°	Vimblastine
3°	Dacarbzin

Infusion order	Medication
VAC	
1°	Vimblastine
2°	Doxorubicin
3°	Cisplatin

Infusion order	Medication
IC	
1°	Irinotecan
2°	Cisplatin

Infusion Speed

Bolus or Push EV	Fast Administration	Within 1minute
Fast EV	Rapid Infusion	Between 1 and 30 minutes
Slow EV	Slow Infusion	Between 30 and 60 minutes
Continuous EV	Slow and Continuous Infusion	Over 60 minutes and continuous
Intermittent EV	Slow Infusion	Over 60 minutes, but not continuous

Drug Administration/Administration Routes

The following guidelines provide a brief commentary on the care required when administering drugs through different routes of administration.

Sublingual drug administration

1.	Place the drug under the patient's tongue and instruct the patient to keep his mouth closed until the drug is completely dissolved;

Observe the patient's reactions;

3.	Guide the patient not to swallow the drug, nor to ingest liquids/food until the drug is completely dissolved;

4.	In case of hypotension, check blood pressure before and 10 minutes after administration;

For incompatibility and continuous solutions, see the stability table available in this manual.

Subcutaneous drug administration

Aspirate with your dominant hand, holding the plunger and gently pulling back to make sure you don't hit a blood vessel;

2.	Observe the patient's reactions; maximum volume: 1.0 (one) ml, and 90° skin angle, paying attention to the maximum dosage for each age;

Application sites: external face of the arm, anterior and posterior, anterolateral face of the thigh, abdominal region (avoid applying in the midline and periumbilical region), apply about 5 cm away from the umbilical scar, it can also be applied in the gluteal, lumbar and infrascapular regions;

If, after the puncture, when aspirating, there is blood return, it means that a vessel was hit, in this case, remove the needle, discard the medication, and prepare another dose for application;

5.   In case of insulin or heparin, do not massage the site;

6.   Heparin. Do not aspirate;

Apply 5cm away from the umbilical scar, ecchymosis or lesions.

8.   For incompatibility and continuous solutions, see the Stability Table available in this manual.

Administration of medication by otologic route

1)   Position the patient with the head of the bed tilted to the side opposite the affected ear to facilitate instillation of the medication;

With your gloved hand, pull the edge of the pinna (helix) upward and backward in the case of an adult patient. In case of a child under 3 years of age, pull the external ear canal downwards and backwards;

Bring the dropper close to the ear canal and instill the medication, avoiding touching the dropper to the patient;

4.   Ask the patient to stay in position for 5 min after instilling the medicine in each ear pinna;

For incompatibility and continuous solutions, see the stability table available in this manual.

Ocular drug administration

For eye drops: gently pull the lower eyelid with the index finger wrapped in gauze, exposing the fundus of the conjunctival sac (instruct the patient to look upwards);

Instill the eye drops in the central region of the conjunctival sac. Avoid touching the dropper (or tube) on the patient's conjunctiva to avoid contaminating the bottle;

Release the lower eyelid, and ask the patient to keep his eyes closed for one minute to promote the contact of the eye drops with the conjunctiva;

4.   Ointment: gently traction the lower eyelid with the index finger wrapped in gauze, exposing the fundus of the conjunctival sac;

Deposit this strip of ointment into the conjunctival sac along the length of the eye;

6.   Remove the excess ointment with gauze; In children or adults who do not open their eyes, apply the eye drops to the inner corner of the eye;

7.   Apply the ointment preferably in the evening if prescribed once a day;

Do not instill the medication directly into the pupil;

9   .Perform ocular hygiene with SF 0.9% and gauze before administering the medication.

For incompatibility and continuous solutions, refer to the stability table available in this manual.

Vaginal drug administration

1.   promote external washing, to favor the contact of the medication with the vaginal mucosa;

2.   the plunger should be introduced about 5 cm into the back wall of the vagina

Remove the applicator and dispose of it in the infectious waste;

4.   Guide the patient to remain lying down (for at least 30 minutes) to favor the permanence of the medication in the vaginal canal;

5.   In the case of an ovule or tablet, the application is similar, using the corresponding applicator;

6.   Apply the medication at night to favor the permanence of the medication in the vaginal canal;

7.   The suppository should be introduced its rounded tip into the back wall of the vagina and about 7.5 to 10 cm;

8.   For incompatibility and continuous solutions, see the Stability Table available in this manual.

Rectal drug administration

1.   In adults and older children, use the index finger to ensure the suppository passes through the internal sphincter about 7.5 cm;

Use xylocaine gel in case of probing;

Inspect the anal area and in case of hemorrhoids or inflamed tissues, do not apply the suppository and report to the doctor;

4.   When retention enema is used (delivery of certain medications) the patient needs to retain the liquid in the rectum or colon for 30 to 60 minutes;

For incompatibility and continuous solutions, see the stability table available in this manual.

Cutaneous (topical) drug administration

Discard the first portion of the ointment;

Place the ointment on the sterile gauze avoiding touching the tip of the tube on the gauze in order not to contaminate it;

Apply in the indicated place with the help of gauze and sterile tweezers, in open wound and integral skin, spread with gloved hand;

4.   Jar: Remove the ointment from the jar using a sterile gauze to avoid contamination of the contents;

5.   Application of lotions and creams: use gloved hand. Before performing any topical application, make sure that the skin is clean and dry, without remnants of previous applications. Exception: aluminum paste do not remove the remainder;

The application should be in the direction of the hair and uniform and in the cephalo-caudal direction;

7.   Shake the lotions before applications to homogenize the ingredients;

8.   For incompatibility and continuous solutions, see the stability table available in this manual.

Administration of liquid medication into the nostrils

1.   sanitize the nostrils;

Bring the dropper close to the nostril and instill the medication;

3.   give a paper towel to the patient to hold next to the nostril and ask him to keep the position for 1 minute, so that the medicine stays in the nose and doesn't run down the face;

4. Guide the patient to inhale deeply to favor the entry of the medication into the nasal cavity; Guide the patient to remain lying down or sitting with the neck hyperextended for 01 minute.

5. the dropper is for individual use

6. For mupirocin application, follow the recommendations of the SCIH;

7. Unconscious patients or children should be positioned with the neck hyperextended for one minute in bed after application of the medication.

8. For incompatibility and continuous solutions, see the stability table available in this manual.

Inhalation therapy (aerosol therapy)

1. Place the medication in the bubbling chamber as prescribed;

2. Place the patient in the "fowler" position to facilitate thoracic expansion during the procedure;

3. Perform airway hygienization, if necessary;

4. Prepare the solution to be administered in the inhaler cup;

Turn on the gas output valve (flow meter to 5 liters) and observe if vaporization is occurring through the inhaler (mist output),

Place the inhalation mask on the face of the patient including nose and mouth;

7- Guide the patient to stay with the mask until the end of inhalation or hold it for him/her in case he/she is dependent on the nursing staff to do so;

Wait for the entire contents of the inhaler cup to evaporate;

Close the flowmeter valve;

Remove the inhaler from the patient's face and keep it protected in a plastic bag according to the SCIH standard;

11. Watch for tachycardia before, during, and after nebulization with bronchodilators;

In case of unconscious/dependent patients, stay by their side until the inhalation is finished;

13. In patients with a tracheostomy, place the mask of the inhaler close to the tracheostomy hole.

Inhalation therapy (aerosol therapy) by respirator circuit (with bubble chamber)

Connect the circuit to the oxygen flow meter;

Connect the respirator circuit adapter between the circuit, the inspiratory pathway, and the bacteriological filter;

Remove the mask from the bubble chamber and connect it to the respirator circuit adapter (at the free outlet);

Open the oxygen flow meter to 5/min (if you have your own respirator circuit, connect it to the device, to its outlet, and turn on the "nebulizer" button);

Wait for the entire contents of the bubbling chamber to evaporate;

6.   Close the oxygen flowmeter (if respirator circuit itself, turn off the "nebulizer" button;

7.   Disconnect the bubble chamber from the respirator circuit adapter;

8.   Protect the inhaler set with a plastic bag and label it with the date;

9.   Keep the inhaler mask in the plastic with its assembly so that it is not lost;

Change the inhaler set every 24 hours or when visibly dirty;

11.   Watch for tachycardia before, during, and after nebulization with bronchodilators.

Administer medication intradermally

Insert the bevel of the needle upwards into the skin at an angle of 15 degrees;

2.   Gently inject the prescribed volume until an orange peel-like papule forms;

3.   Observe the patient and reactions at the application site (more or less 30 minutes);

4.   Internationally standardized site of BCG application: lower insertion area of the deltoid muscle of the right arm;

Ventral side of the forearm (region with little pigmentation, poor hair, easy access for reading the results of sensitivity tests and little superficial vascularity);

6.   Prior antisepsis of ID injections or local compression after application with cotton soaked in antiseptic solution is not recommended with the skin and drug, which may mask sensitivity reactions and inactivate or decrease the potency of the drug;

7.   Maximum volume: 0.5 ml;

8.   PPD tests are read after 24 or 48 to 72 hours. During this period you may not administer any medication to the limb used for the test, nor should you measure BP or administer serum to it;

If you apply more than one ID injection, the distance between them must be 5 cm;

10.   Advise the patient not to scratch or rub the injection site;

11.   If any sign of allergic reaction occurs (dyspnea, tachycardia, bradycardia, etc.) immediately notify the doctor.

12.   For incompatibility and continuous solutions, see the Stability Table available in this manual.

<u>Oral/enteral medication administration</u>

1.   take the medicine out of its package, place it in the cup and offer it to the patient, and offer 01 pill at a time;

For liquid medication: pour the medication into the cup or aspirate with the syringe without contaminating the bottle;

3.   When placing the medicine in the cup, pour the liquid from the opposite side of the label;

Take the measurement in the cup (you must keep it at eye level);

5.   Offer pills first, and in sequence lozenges, capsules, pills, liquids, and lastly sublingual medications;

6.   If the tablet is not grooved, it cannot be broken (report to the pharmacy);

7.   No medication from illegible bottles or labels may be administered;

For tube administration, follow good enteral nutrition practice protocol.

9.   Do not leave medication on the patient's bedside table;

Observe the patient's level of consciousness/swallowing ability before offering medication.

9.   For incompatibility and continuous solutions, see the Stability Table available in this manual.

<u>Intramuscular (IM) administration of medication</u>

1.   perform antisepsis in a circular fashion from inside to outside, starting from the chosen point;

Make sure there is no air inside the syringe;

Insert the needle with the bevel on the side and inject the medication;

Insert the syringe and aspirate, if blood returns, remove the needle and prepare a new medication in a new syringe and needle (justify in the chart);

Remove the needle and compress the site with dry absorbent cotton;

Do not apply IM injection in immobile limbs, inflamed or edematous site, birthmarks, scar tissue, patients with coagulation disorders and patients with acute myocardial infarction, except with written medical authorization.

For incompatibility and continuous solutions, refer to the stability table available in this manual.

<u>Intravenous (IV) medication administration</u>

General Orientations

1.   Verify that the patient has previous access;

Provide venous access in case it is not available (according to the venipuncture technique);

In cases of care for a patient in emergency situations, if the patient presents clinical conditions that suggest a longer period of observation or even hospitalization, after puncturing the vein for administration of a drug (e.g. analgesic), maintain the venous access route (salinization) to avoid repuncture;

4.   Heparinization will be used only in double lumen catheter and fully implanted catheter;

5.   Do not aspirate the venous catheter before administration of the medication;

Wash the venous access with SF0.9% or ABD before and after administration of the medication;

7.   In case of slow infusion medication with syringe, close the three-way stopcock for the other solutions (consult the physician beforehand in case of continuous medication and request written authorization);

When several drugs are administered simultaneously in the same access, the one with the lowest flow rate will be farthest from the access;

9-   When you are going to administer a medication in a venous access in which you are infusing a solution and it cannot be interrupted, it is necessary to puncture   another venous access to administer the medication or, in extreme cases of difficult venous puncture, to have the physician's written authorization to administer the medication in the same access as the incompatible solution;

Do not let air into the infusion line during infusion;

11.   Regarding the expiration date of the venous access (96h) for children and elderly, it may remain after the deadline, and should be rigorously evaluated (signs of phlebitis, impaired perfusion) due to the difficulty of repuncture;

12.   For incompatibility and continuous solutions, see the Stability Table available in this manual.

Intravenous (IV) drug administration by side injector

1.   rub cotton soaked in 70% alcohol for 30 seconds 3 consecutive times on the injector rubber;

2.   clamp the equipment;

Puncture the injector;

Inject the medication;

Remove the syringe with needle;

6.   unclamp the equipment;

Do not let air into the infusion line during infusion;

8.   For incompatibility and continuous solutions, see the stability table available in this manual.

Intravenous medication administration (iv) bolus medication incompatible with primary course solution

1.   Perform disinfection of the three-way stopcock;

Close the three-way stopcock for the solution in progress;

Wash the access with 0.9% saline solution or ABD, according to the lumen of the catheter;

Inject the medication;

Rinse the access again;

Open the three-way stopcock for the solution;

7.   Keep the three-way stopcock always protected with its cap;

8.   For incompatibility and continuous solutions, see the stability table available in this manual.

<u>Drug administration by intravenous (iv) infusion in y (compatible solutions).</u>

1. Perform disinfection of the three-way stopcock;

Install the medication line in the three-way tap outlet closest to the venous access;

Control the dripping, observing the medical prescription;

At the end: open the three-way stopcock for other solutions;

Disconnect the medication line and protect its extremity with its cap;

Protect the three-way stopcock with the cap;

For incompatibility and continuous solutions, refer to the stability table available in this manual.

<u>Administer medication by intravenous (iv) burette infusion (microfix)</u>

Check the microfix label with the medication label;

2. rub the cotton with 70% alcohol in the injector;

Add the diluent (SF 0.9% or SGI5%) to the microfix;

Inject the medication into the microfix;

Fill the container with the solution, observing the level and opening the forceps slowly, observing for the presence of air;

6. Close the IV clamp and keep it connected to the microfix;

7. In the case of newborn medication, fill the entire microfix syringe with the prescribed solution and add the medication into the side injector.

Then, connect the microfix IV line to the venous access and allow the medication to be infused until the infusion stops. At this moment, fill the burette with 10 ml of the prescribed solution and open the clamp waiting, at the bedside, for the rest of the medication to be infused;

Disconnect the line from the venous access, protect the end of the line, and salinize the access;

In cases of dosages in which a volume greater than 10 ml is required for dilution of the medication, this volume must be measured in the burette with the line previously filled with the prescribed diluent. The medication will be added into the burette through the silicone device in the upper part of the Microfix;

In cases of intravenous devices: observe the conditions of the puncture site, check for the presence of signs of inflammation and secretions, use aseptic technique for handling and control the date of puncture (96 hours);

12.   In case of slow infusion medication with syringe, close the three-way stopcock for the other solutions (consult your physician beforehand in case of continuous medication);

Identify one microfix for each medication and do not let air into the IV line during infusion;

14.   The use of Microfix will be recommended when it is impossible to administer the bolus medication slowly (20 to 30 minutes) in a syringe pump;

15.   For incompatibility and continuous solutions, see the Stability Table available in this manual.

<u>Aspirate medication in ampoule or vial</u>

Aspirate medicine in ampoules:

1.   Gather the material;

2.   wash your hands;

Disinfect the neck of the ampoule with cotton soaked in 70% alcohol;

4.   Break the ampoule protecting the neck with dry cotton balls to avoid injuring your hands;

Remove the needle protector, placing it in the syringe packaging;

Position the ampoule between the index and middle fingers of the non-dominant hand;

Insert the needle into the ampoule, without touching the neck of the ampoule, with the bevel facing down to avoid contamination of the needle and to facilitate aspiration;

Aspirate the medication without contaminating the syringe plunger;

Support the plunger with your non-dominant hand and position the syringe vertically with the needle up and protected by its cap;

10.   Remove the air from inside the syringe by pushing the plunger gently until the liquid column reaches the needle barrel;

11.   Change the needle (40X12) for one suitable for the application;

12.   place the syringe in the tray with the identification label on the outside of its package, protect the plunger with its package and the needle with its cap.

 Aspirate medication into vial:

13.   Gather the material;

14. Wash your hands or rub them with alcohol gel for 15 seconds in the absence of apparent dirt;

Remove the central part of the protection cover with scissors and disinfect it with cotton soaked in 70% alcohol;

Aspirate the diluent in the necessary amount;

Insert the needle into the vial, perforating the rubber stopper;

Inject the diluent slowly into the wall of the vial and remove the needle, protecting it with the cap to avoid contamination;

19. Homogenize the contents with rotary movements, slowly taking care that the medication does not foam;

20. Aspirate the solution with the syringe;

Discard the needle used for aspiration and connect the appropriate needle for the application (in case the drug is aspirated with a 40x12 needle);

Place the syringe in the tray with the identification label on the package (externally), protect the plunger with the package itself and the needle with its cap.

Cautions when administering medications

1. Refuse to administer medication if the prescription is illegible, confusing or obscure;

2. Clarify a confusing prescription rather than trying to interpret it;

3. Obtain clarification from the prescribing physician and, if he or she cannot be found, from the chief of clinic;

4. Contact the clinical director as a last resort;

5. Record in the nursing evolution that the medication was not administered, its reason, and to whom it was communicated in case you are not sure that it should be administered;

6. Circulate on the prescription the time that the medication was not administered and sign it;

7. Know what drug allergies would be experienced by the patient;

8. Identify the medications that the patient continuously uses and communicate to the physician in order to predict and avoid drug interactions;

9. Verify if the patient is using medication brought from home and communicate it to the physician. Also inform the pharmacist, proceeding as described in the chapter "Medication brought by the patient".

<u>**Management when a patient refuses medication**</u>

Inform the patient about his or her medical condition and the possible results of his or her refusal;

2.   Inform the nurse and the doctor;

Record the refusal in the nursing evolution;

4.   Fill out the patient's medication refusal form;

5.   Identify the form with the patient's full name and the name of the medications;

6.   collect the signatures of the witnesses;

7.   collect the signature of the patient or guardian;

Sign, date, and stamp;

9.   In the case of illiterate patients or those unable to sign, the patient's fingerprints will be taken.

<u>**Medication Checking**</u>

1.   Check the medication immediately after its administration;

2.   Mark with a dash (/) over the time when the medication is administered;

3.   Then sign legibly your first name (not your last name);

4.   Stamp at the end of the prescription (one stamp per shift);

Register in the nursing evolution the medications that were administered in the emergency room and evolve any intercurrence as well as its expected effects.

<u>**Management of cytostatic extravasation**</u>

Extravasation is the escape of a drug from a blood vessel into the surrounding tissues. The morbidity depends on the drug, the amount extravasated and its concentration, the location of the extravasation, the patient's condition, and the interval between the event and its recognition and treatment.

Vesicant drugs are those that cause severe irritation with vesicle formation and tissue destruction when infiltrated outside the blood vessel.

Irritant drugs cause less intense skin reaction when extravasated: pain and burning without tissue necrosis or vesicle formation.

Non Vesicants	Irritants	Vesicants
Asparaginase	Bortezomib	Dactinomycin
Bleomycin	Carmustina	Daunorrubicin
Carboplatin	Cisplatin	Doxorubicin
Cyclophosphamide	Dacarbazine	Epirubicin
Cytarabine	Docetaxel	Mitomycin
Fludarabine	Liposomal doxorubicin	Mitoxantrone
Diluted Fluoruracil	Etoposide	Paclitaxel
Ifosfamide	Undiluted Fluoruracil	Vimblastine
Irinotecan	Gencitabine	Vincristine
Methotrexate	Oxaliplatin	Vinorelbine
Pemetrexede		
Topotecan		

Reference: Extravasation of cytotoxic agents, 2nd edition Springer-verlag Wien New York
(Material - Oncologia Sandoz)

<u>Signs and symptoms of extravasation</u>

They can occur immediately or a few days or weeks after application.

The immediate reactions are: burning, local discomfort and erythema.

The late reactions are pain, edema, induration, ulceration, vesicles, necrosis, cellulitis, and inflammation.

<u>**Basic measures in case of extravasation**</u>

Immediately stop the infusion and keep the needle in place.

2)   connect a syringe to the device and aspirate the residual medication in the device and, if possible, part of the extravasated medication into the tissues

Apply the recommended antidote, if indicated (see Antidotes)

Remove the needle and raise the limb above the level of the heart.

5.   For all drugs, with the exception of the vinca alkaloids (vincristine, vimblastine, and vinorelbine) and epipodophyllotoxins (etoposide), the application of ice or cold compresses for 15 to 20 minutes at least four times a day for the first 24 to 48 hours is recommended.

Avoid direct manual pressure on the affected area.

7.   Photograph the affected area for documentation and follow-up.

Notify the physician and the nurse with experience in extravasation for adequate registration and follow-up. The following data are important: date and time, type of needle and gauge, location, drug (s) administered and sequence, amount extravasated, signs and symptoms presented, treatment performed, and signature of the nurse in charge.

<u>**Antidotes**</u>

Antidotes should be administered immediately after infiltration, through the same needle, after aspiration of the largest possible amount of infiltrated drug or subcutaneously, if the needle has already been withdrawn. The objective is to limit the local inflammation process, inactivate the remaining drug, and quickly remove it from the site. Its use must be prescribed by the physician or authorized by protocol defined by the institution.

AGENT/CLASS	LOCAL ANIMAL RECOMMENDED	SPECIAL PROCEDURE
Anthracyclines • Doxorubicin • Daunorrubicin	Cold compresses	Apply immediately for 30 to 60 minutes, then alternate every 15 minutes for 1 day. Apply 1,5mL to the site of the extravasation every 6h for 14 days. Leave the place ventilated, do not cover.
Vinca Alkaloids • Vimblastine • Vincristine • Vinorelbine	Warm compresses Hyaluronidase	Apply warm compresses immediately for 30 to 60 minutes, then alternate every 15 minutes for 1 day. Mix 150U of hyaluronidase with 1-3Ml of 0.9% saline solution. Inject the hyaluronidase through the I.V. catheter cannula, being 1mL for each 1mL extravasated. After that, inject the antidote around the site of extravasation
Epinodofilotoxins • Etoposide • Teniposido	Warm compresses Hyaluronidase	Apply warm compresses immediately for 30 to 60 minutes, then alternate every 15 minutes for 1 day. Mix 150U of hyaluronidase with 1-3mL of 0.9% saline solution. Inject the hyaluronidase through the I.V. catheter cannula, being 1mL for each 1mL extravasated. After that, inject the antidote around the site of extravasation.
Taxanos • Paclitaxel • Docetaxel	Ice packs Hyaluronidase	Apply the ice packs for 15 to 20 minutes at least 4 times a day for the first 24 hours. Mix 300U of hyaluronidase with 3mL of 0.9% saline solution. Inject the hyaluronidase through the I.V. catheter cannula, being 1mL for each 1mL extravasated. After that, inject the antidote around the site of extravasation.

Antidotes used in case of extravasation of antineoplastic drugs.

<u>**Conduct in case of spill of cytostatics in the environment**</u>

In case of spillage of cytostatics, use the "Spill Kit", available in the sector. The kit contains the following items:

- 2 pairs of procedure gloves

- 1 disposable, waterproof apron

- 2 absorbent pads

- 1 mask with active carbon filter

- 1 goggle

- 1 plastic bag identified as toxic waste

. 1 almotól of liquid soap

The kit is to be used in case of vial drop or cytostatic drug spill, and should be used according to "SOP for antineoplastic drug spills".

If you have any questions, please contact the Chemotherapy sector through extension 2106 or e-mail viviannie@santacasamontesclaros.com.br.

<u>**Management of side effects**</u>

Nausea and vomiting

The purpose of cancer treatment is to cure or relieve the symptoms of the disease. Drug treatments (chemotherapy, targeted therapy, hormone therapy), surgery, and radiation therapy can cause side effects that vary from patient to patient depending on multiple factors, and may differ in intensity and duration. Some patients may experience more severe side effects, others more mild, or no side effects at all. If you experience any side effects due to the treatment you are undergoing, consult your doctor immediately to receive the necessary guidance for your case. Some types of chemotherapy can cause nausea and vomiting, which can occur during treatment, after or days after the administration of the chemo. Mild nausea and vomiting can be very uncomfortable, but usually does not cause serious problems. Persistent vomiting can lead to dehydration, hydro-electrolyte imbalance, weight loss, and decreased general condition, all of which may require discontinuation of treatment.

Causes

Nausea and vomiting in people undergoing cancer treatment can be caused by:

- Radiation therapy to the brain, spinal cord, abdomen, pelvis, or whole body.
- Brain metastasis.
- Obstructed bowel.
- Water-electrolyte imbalance.
- Infections or bleeding in the gastrointestinal system.
- Heart disease.
- Medications.

Acute vomiting is vomiting that occurs within the first 24 hours after treatment. Late vomiting may occur up to two or more days after treatment.

People who are more likely to experience chemoinduced nausea and vomiting are:

- People who have already vomited after cancer treatment.
- People who are prone to motion sickness.
- People who get anxious before treatment.
- People under the age of 50, especially women.

Prevention and Management

Whenever possible, it is best to prevent nausea and vomiting. There are many medications available to help reduce or stop vomiting, such as antiemetics that can be prescribed before treatment begins. Some behavioral treatments, such as relaxation and mentalization, can help control nausea and vomiting.

Tips

- One way to prevent vomiting is to avoid nausea; to do this, it is recommended that you eat easily digestible foods and drinks.
- Plan your meals, some people feel better when they eat before chemotherapy, others prefer not to eat anything, this is very variable, however you should wait at least an hour after chemotherapy before you can have any food or drink.
- Eat small meals, preferably 5 to 6 a day. Do not drink too much liquid before or during meals, and do not lie down immediately after eating.

- Consume warm, cool foods and drinks, wait for hot foods and drinks to cool down, and avoid carbonated beverages.
- Avoid strong foods and drinks such as coffee, fish, onions, garlic, or very hot foods, as these can trigger nausea and therefore vomiting.
- Before chemotherapy begins, it is good to relax. Try to do activities that you enjoy, for example, meditate, read a book, or listen to music. This will make you feel less nauseous.
- Evaluate with your doctor the antiemetic medications, see if they are working or not. Tell your doctor if you have experienced nausea and vomiting and for how long, mentioning if you vomited right after eating something, drinking something, or if it was when you took some medicine.

Depression

The purpose of cancer treatment is to cure or relieve the symptoms of the disease. Drug treatments (chemotherapy, targeted therapy, hormone therapy), surgery, and radiation therapy can cause side effects that vary from patient to patient depending on multiple factors, and may differ in intensity and duration. Some patients may experience more severe side effects, others more mild, or no side effects at all. In case you experience any side effects due to the treatment you are undergoing, consult your doctor immediately to receive the necessary guidance for your case. Depression can be common in people with cancer, but is not often diagnosed. However, this does not mean that all people with cancer have depression.

Symptoms

The two most common symptoms of depression are depressed mood and loss of interest in normal activities. Other symptoms of depression include:

- Insomnia or other sleep disorders.
- Variation in weight.
- Change in appetite.
- Fatigue and loss of energy.
- Feelings of irritability or agitation.
- Feelings of worthlessness or guilt.
- Feelings of hopelessness or helplessness.

- Thoughts of self-injury or suicide.
- Preoccupation with death.
- Difficulty in concentrating.
- Social regression.
- Crying fits.
- Feeling slow.

Generally, if a person has a depressed mood or a loss of interest in activities that he or she previously enjoyed, and at least four of the symptoms mentioned above more than twice a week, it is recommended that they talk to their doctor about the possibility of treatment.

Risk Factors and Diagnosis

They can increase the likelihood that a patient will experience depression:

- History of depression prior to cancer diagnosis.
- History of alcoholism or drug abuse.
- Increased physical weakness or discomfort caused by cancer.
- Pain out of control.
- Medication.
- Advanced cancer.
- Imbalances of calcium, sodium, potassium, or vitamin B12.
- Other nutritional problems.
- Neurological difficulties.
- Hyperthyroidism or hypothyroidism.

Doctors may perform a number of tests to diagnose depression, including questions about behavior, feelings, and thoughts.

Depression Management and Treatment

Almost all types of depression are treatable. Treatment for depression helps the cancer patient to manage the disease, and often involves psychological treatment with antidepressant medication. The focus of psychological treatment is on increasing coping and problem-solving skills. The most common methods include individual psychotherapy and cognitive behavioral therapy. In addition, cancer patient support groups may be helpful for some people with cancer who have depression.

Because out-of-control pain is related to depression, it is important that patients seek help for pain management and other symptoms, such as fatigue.

Medications

The doctor may recommend antidepressants. Most antidepressants treat depression by changing the brain chemistry that may be the cause of depression. If you and your doctor decide that medication is the next step, keep this in mind:

- Different types of antidepressants have different side effects, including sexual, nausea, insomnia, dry mouth, or heart problems. Others may improve anxiety or have a faster effect. However, side effects can usually be managed by adjusting the dose or changing the medication.
- Many people with cancer take many different medications, which can interact and interfere with the effectiveness of another, causing harm. Always tell your doctor about all the medications you are using, including medicinal therapies.
- Although almost 15% to 25% of cancer patients have depression, only 2% are treated with antidepressants.

Dry Mouth

The purpose of cancer treatment is to cure or relieve the symptoms of the disease. Drug treatments (chemotherapy, targeted therapy, hormone therapy), surgery, and radiation therapy can cause side effects that vary from patient to patient depending on multiple factors, and may differ in intensity and duration. Some patients may experience more severe side effects, others more mild, or no side effects at all. In case you experience any side effects due to the treatment you are undergoing, consult your physician immediately to receive the necessary guidance for your case. Dry mouth occurs when the salivary glands do not produce enough saliva to keep the mouth moist. Since saliva is needed for chewing, swallowing, tasting, and speaking, these activities can become more difficult.

Causes

Dry mouth can be caused by chemotherapy or radiation therapy, which damage the salivary glands. Dry mouth caused by chemotherapy makes saliva thicker, causing a dry feeling, which is usually temporary and reverses within two to eight weeks after treatment ends.

Radiation therapy of the head and neck region can also cause dry mouth. After radiotherapy treatment ends it can take six months or more for the salivary glands to begin producing saliva again. Despite some improvement patients may experience dryness during the first year after radiotherapy treatment, and many will continue to have some level of dryness indefinitely, especially if the radiotherapy was directed at the salivary glands.

Dry and sore mouth can also be caused when a bone marrow transplant is performed. In addition, some types of medications, including antidepressants, diuretics and painkillers, can cause dry mouth. Dry mouth can also be the result of a mouth infection or dehydration.

Signs and Symptoms

- Dry, unpleasant sensation in the mouth.
- Dense, fibrous saliva.
- Pain or burning sensation in the mouth or on the tongue.
- Cracks in the lips or corners of the mouth.
- Dry, stiff tongue.
- Difficulty chewing, tasting, or swallowing.
- Difficulty speaking.
- Difficulty wearing dentures.
- Ulcers or infections in the mouth.
- Dental caries.

Associated Problems

In addition to difficulty eating and speaking, dry mouth can cause dental problems. Saliva helps maintain the balance of bacteria in the mouth and protects against infection and tooth decay. Without enough saliva, bacteria and other organisms can grow very quickly in the mouth, causing infections and sores. Saliva washes away acids and food particles left in the mouth after eating. Therefore, a lack of saliva can cause tooth decay and gum disease.

Management

Although dry mouth cannot be prevented, some treatments can help. Patients who have radiation therapy to the head or neck may have to use a radioprotective medication, which reduces the severity of dry mouth.

Some tips to help prevent dry mouth and dental problems:

- Go to the dentist before starting treatment, radiotherapy or chemotherapy, to check the health of your mouth and teeth.
- Brush your teeth at least four times a day with a soft-bristled brush and fluoride toothpaste.
- Gently floss once a day.
- Rinse your mouth four to six times a day, especially after meals, with baking soda solution.
- Drink small sips of water throughout the day and use artificial saliva to moisten the mouth.
- Chew sugarless gum or suck on sugarless candy to increase saliva flow.
- Avoid mouthrinses with dental products containing alcohol.
- Some dentists prescribe the use of a fluoride gel to increase saliva production.

Food Tips

- Drink at least eight glasses of water a day.
- Avoid alcoholic and caffeinated beverages and acidic juices.
- Eat soft, moist, cold, or room temperature foods.
- Moisten dry food with broth, sauces, butter or milk.
- Avoid dry, rough, or hard foods.
- Avoid acidic or spicy foods.
- Do not smoke or chew tobacco.
- Avoid sticky foods and sugary drinks.

Fatigue

The purpose of cancer treatment is to cure or relieve the symptoms of the disease. Drug treatments (chemotherapy, targeted therapy, hormone therapy), surgery, and radiation therapy can cause side effects that vary from patient to patient depending on multiple factors, and may differ in intensity and duration. Some patients may experience more severe side effects, others more mild, or no side effects at all. In case you experience any side effects due to the treatment you are undergoing, consult your doctor immediately to receive the necessary guidance for your case. Cancer-related fatigue is a persistent feeling of tiredness or exhaustion. People who experience fatigue during treatment often say that even a small effort, such as walking indoors, can be very difficult. Fatigue can seriously affect a patient's daily activities, including his or her ability to work and relate to family and friends or to socialize. Fatigue can lead people to avoid or skip steps in treatment and even affect their desire to live.

Fatigue may arise after treatment in the following circumstances:

- A few days after chemotherapy treatment.
- A few weeks after the start of radiotherapy treatment.
- After treatment with immunotherapy.

Sometimes other conditions can contribute to fatigue, including pain, depression, or insomnia.

Diagnosis

It is important to tell your doctor if you are experiencing fatigue. He or she will order a blood test to determine if you have anemia or another condition that may be causing the symptom.

Fatigue Management

- Exercise regularly.
- Conserve your energy.
- Get treatment for depression, pain, sleep disorders, or other conditions that may be associated with fatigue.

Alopecia

The purpose of cancer treatment is to cure or relieve the symptoms of the disease. Drug treatments (chemotherapy, targeted therapy, hormone therapy), surgery, and radiation therapy can cause side effects that vary from patient to patient depending on multiple factors, and may differ in intensity and duration. Some patients may experience more severe side effects, others more mild, or no side effects at all. If you experience any side effects due to the treatment you are undergoing, consult your doctor immediately to receive the necessary guidance for your case. One of the side effects of radiotherapy and chemotherapy treatments is hair loss (alopecia), which can occur all over the body, including the head, face, arms, legs, armpits, and pubic area.

Hair can fall out all at once, or gradually. Hair loss is often a challenging experience, both psychologically and emotionally, as it affects self-image and quality of life. However, hair loss is temporary, and hair will grow back after treatment is over.

Causes

Radiotherapy and chemotherapy cause hair loss by damaging the hair follicles responsible for hair growth.

Chemotherapy - Not all chemotherapy treatments cause hair loss, it all depends on the type of drugs used. When hair loss does occur, it is generally not immediate, and the amount of hair loss varies from person to person, even among those taking the same medication. Hair loss usually occurs after the first few weeks or cycles of chemotherapy and tends to increase as treatment continues. With the end of chemotherapy, the hair regrows back.

Radiotherapy - Radiotherapy affects only the hair in the regions within the irradiated area, and depends on the radiation dose. However, for high doses of radiation, hair loss is permanent.

Management

In some cases, hair loss due to cancer treatment is not prevented or treated with stimulants, solutions, or special shampoos. Therefore, learning how to deal with hair loss before it occurs helps the patient to prepare for this change in appearance. Talking about feelings with a therapist, with someone who has gone through a similar experience, with a family member or friend can provide some comfort. Also, when hair loss is inevitable, this should be talked about with family members, friends, and especially children before it occurs.

Some people prefer to cut their hair shorter before treatment begins, which makes the loss less traumatic.

Hair and Scalp Care

- Choose a mild shampoo to cleanse the hair and scalp.
- Use a soft hair brush to tidy up the remaining hair.
- Use sunscreen on your scalp when outdoors.
- Cover your head during the colder months to prevent loss of body heat.
- Avoid drying your hair at high temperatures.
- Avoid the use of chemicals.
- Avoid doing a perm.
- Use pillowcases with soft fabrics.

Wigs and Hairpieces

- Choose a wig or applique before hair loss, if you prefer similar to the type and color of your original hair.
- When purchasing a wig make sure that it is comfortable and will not irritate the scalp.

Growing Hair Care

Hair begins to grow back within 2 to 3 months after chemotherapy ends, and full hair growth sometimes takes 6 to 12 months. Temporarily, the texture and color of the new hair may be different from your hair before the fall, but the pigment cells regenerate spontaneously, and soon your hair returns to its original color. Some care must be taken during hair growth:

- Try to wash your hair only twice a week.
- Massage the scalp to remove dry skin.
- Limit the amount of brushing, clipping, and blow-drying at high temperatures. The new hair will initially be much finer and more prone to breakage than the original hair.

- Avoid curling or straightening your hair with chemicals until it has reached at least 3 cm in length.
- Avoid perming and coloring for at least three months after the end of the treatment.

Tips

Before you start chemotherapy, talk to your doctor about the side effects you may face:

- Cut your hair, as this will give you a greater sense of control over hair loss and makes it easier to manage hair loss.
- If you prefer to wear a wig, buy one while you still have hair. Choose one in a similar shade to your hair that is comfortable and won't hurt your scalp.
- Take care when washing your head, use a mild shampoo, dry your head with a soft towel and with gentle movements, do not rub.
- Do not use items or products that can hurt your scalp such as electric hair dryers, hair dyes, or perming products.

After hair loss it is recommended that you:

- Protect your head, especially your scalp, which may be sensitive, with a hat, turban, or headscarf.
- Do not stay in environments with very low or very high temperatures. Always use a sunblock to protect your scalp.
- When you go to sleep use a pillow with a satin pillowcase, this type of fabric creates less friction than a cotton fabric, and can be more comfortable to sleep on.

Hand-Foot Syndrome

The purpose of cancer treatment is to cure or relieve the symptoms of the disease. Drug treatments (chemotherapy, targeted therapy, hormone therapy), surgery, and radiation therapy can cause side effects that vary from patient to patient depending on multiple factors, and may differ in intensity and duration. Some patients may experience more severe side effects, others more mild, or no side effects at all. In case you experience any side effects due to the treatment you are undergoing, consult your doctor immediately to receive the necessary guidance for your case. Hand-foot syndrome is a side effect of some types of chemotherapy, which causes redness, swelling, and pain in the palms of the hands or soles of the feet.

Although less common, hand-foot syndrome can also occur in other areas such as knees and elbows.

Symptoms

Moderate hand-foot syndrome can present symptoms such as:

- Redness.
- Swelling.
- Tingling or burning sensation.

Severe symptoms of hand-foot syndrome include:

- Cracking or peeling of the skin.
- Blisters, ulcers, or sores on the skin.
- Severe pain.
- Difficulty walking or using your hands.

Treatment

If you develop severe hand-foot syndrome your doctor may reduce the dose of chemotherapy or change your treatment regimen. If necessary, your doctor will temporarily stop chemotherapy until your symptoms improve.

Medications that can be used to treat hand-foot syndrome are:

- Corticosteroids, to reduce inflammation.
- Vitamin B6, to help decrease the symptoms.
- Painkillers, to relieve pain.

Prevention

Prevention of symptoms focuses on avoiding friction and heat, which make symptoms worse. Recommendations for symptom control and prevention of hand-foot syndrome include:

- Limit exposure of hands and feet to hot water when washing dishes or bathing.
- Take cold or warm baths.
- Avoid exposure to heat sources such as saunas and the sun.

- Avoid activities that cause unnecessary force or friction on the feet, such as running, aerobics, and long walks.
- Avoid contact with chemicals used in detergents or household cleaning products.
- Avoid the use of rubber gloves for cleaning with hot water.
- Avoid using household tools or utensils that require hand pressure against a hard, rough surface, such as garden tools, knives, or screwdrivers.

Other recommendations include:

- Cool the hands and feet with cold compresses or ice packs for 20 minutes.
- Elevate your hands and feet when sitting or lying down.
- Dry the skin carefully after bathing.
- Gently apply creams to keep the hands moist.
- Avoid rubbing or massaging the hands and feet.
- Wear comfortable, loose shoes and clothes.

POP's

Related to Clinical Pharmacy

Prescription analysis: Analyze prescription for clinical protocol.

- Analyze the prescription as to the clinical protocol: indication, dose, frequency, route of administration, drug interactions (pharmacokinetic and pharmacodynamic), drug-food interactions, and incompatibilities;
- If any PRM occurs, analyze the patient's entire clinical history and if any intervention is required, contact the prescribing physician and the multidisciplinary team involved and perform the observations;
- After reviewing the prescription, validate with stamp and signature.

Oncologic and Hematologic Pharmaceutical Care: Perform Pharmaceutical Care

- Guide patients when delivering oral chemotherapeutic and immunotherapeutic drugs, as to how to store and administer them (in order to avoid mistakenly taking the drugs);

- Deliver the orientation booklet for oral chemotherapeutic and immunotherapeutic drugs and formalize the orientation in the patient's chart.

Prescription Fulfillment: Fulfill prescriptions and requests/Realize Pharmacoeconomics.

- Upon receipt and review of the prescription, the entire prescription must be filled as requested;
- Items must be passed through the reader (ensuring traceability);
- You must enter the MGES system, click on the ATTEND REQUEST shortcut, put in the request number or prescription number, click on CONFIRM PRODUCTS, and start passing the products requested by the reader according to the medical prescription;
- Close the write-off after all items entered in the patient's account are completed;
- Dispense the typed items to Oncology Pharmacist.

Dispensing pre-chemotherapy and chemotherapy for nursing: Dispensing pre-chemotherapy and chemotherapy for nursing

- After handling according to SOP DFIN/QUIM/006, seal the chemotherapy in a plastic bag and place it in the patient's tray;
- Place the tray with all prescription medication on the pass-trought so that nursing can pick it up and forward it to the chemotherapy room, according to process interaction between oncology nursing and oncology pharmacy.

Pharmacovigilance: Perform pharmacovigilance.

- Follow up on patients with a history of drug allergy referred to the Oncology Pharmacy through medical triage/consultation (To avoid administering to the patient a drug that he or she is allergic to);
- To monitor and report in the SAS system and via email to the Pharmacovigilance Committee, according to the interaction process between Hospital Pharmacy and Oncology Pharmacy, possible ADRs identified in oncology/hematology patients, evidenced during chemotherapy treatment;

- To follow up and notify via email the Pharmacovigilance Committee and the Hospital Standardization Committee (centralized in the purchasing sector), according to the interaction process between the Hospital Pharmacy and Oncology Pharmacy, the quality deviations of medical/hospital materials.

Receiving and storing hospital supplies and medicines: Receiving and storing hospital supplies and medicines.

- The technician/trainee must check all hospital supplies and medications for quantity, lot, and expiration date using the transfer sheet;
- After checking the items, the technician/trainee must store them in their respective locations (locations are already identified).

Medication Reconciliation: Performing Medication Reconciliation

- You should go to the patient's inpatient/ambulatory ward or caretaker and ask them if they use medications at home and advise them on how to use them at home (if the patient is an outpatient) or in the hospital (if the patient is an inpatient);
- Formalize in the patient's chart the medication reconciliation, sign and stamp it.

POP's

Related to Chemotherapeutic Pharmacotechnology and Hospital Pharmacy

Technique for cleaning up after a cytostatic drug (chemotherapy) spill: Minimize the risk of exposure to chemotherapeutic agents. Properly clean up the area where the cytostatic drug spill occurred.

- Communicate to the assistance team present about the accident and associated risks;
- Request their removal from the site, if possible;
- Identify the spill area and restrict access to it;
- Avoid contact between the drug and the skin and/or mucous membranes;
- Use the kit available in the area where the spill occurred;
- Wear PPEs (contained in the kit) to perform the cleaning of the site.Remember to use two procedure gloves (one on top of the other);

- Limit the spill area with absorbent pads:

  - powders should be collected with absorbent pads moistened with liquid soap.

  -liquids should be collected with dry absorbent pads.

- Clean the area with concentrated liquid soap always from the outside in, to avoid spreading the spill further.

- Collect the fragments, compresses used, and dispose of them in the reinforced plastic bag (2 overlapping bags) of infectious waste contained in the kit.

- Remove the first pair of gloves, discard them in the infectious waste bag, remove the other PPE's (mask, apron) and the last pair of gloves, tie the bag with two knots, taking care not to inhale during the act.

- Identify the waste bag as ``CHEMICAL/CHEMIOTHERAPY WASTE.

- Sanitize your hands immediately after the procedure, according to SOP DTAS/SCIH/021.

- Fill out the proper form contained in the KIT and notify the oncology service pharmacist of the accident. Ext. 2106.

Changing the laminar flow chamber pre-filter: Preserve the quality of the absolute filter in the laminar flow chamber.

- Remove the protective support from the pre-filter inlet in the Laminar Flow cabin;

- Remove the old pre-filter and pack it first in a black bag and then in the infectious waste bag;

- Place the new pre-filter in the cabin, paying attention to the correct position of the pre-filter as directed by the equipment itself (airflow direction arrows);

- Reposition the protective cabin support;

- Forward the old pre-filter for disposal;

- Record the date of the change and sign the registration map.

Completing the chemotherapy label for outpatients and inpatients: Ensure that the drug to be prepared is in the correct dose, concentration, and diluent; ensure that patient identification information is correct; ensure physicochemical stability of the drugs.

- Fill out the compulsory information on the label: full name of the patient; prescribed drug and dose; prescribed diluent and volume; volume corresponding to the prescribed dose; total volume contained in the vial; infusion speed; stability after dilution; date and time of preparation; batch of drug used; signatures of the person responsible for the preparation and for making the label.

Sanitization of the medication refrigerator: Ensure sanitization of the chemotherapy dilution center refrigerator.

- Remove the medication from the refrigerator and pack it in a temperature-controlled thermal box with a maximum and minimum thermometer.
- Clean the inside of the refrigerator with a cloth pad moistened with a little liquid soap;
- With a new pad moistened with water, remove the excess liquid soap;
- With a new compress soaked in 70% alcohol, dry the inside of the refrigerator;
- Close the refrigerator and wait until the internal temperature is between 2 and 8°c;
- Return the medicines to the inside of the refrigerator;
- Record the procedure on the daily refrigerator temperature log chart and sign on the corresponding date.

Handling antineoplastic drugs: Prepare antineoplastic medication in a dose as prescribed by the physician in order to ensure its sterility; ensure the safety of the manipulator in accordance with NR 32 of ANVISA.

- Turn on the CBS 30 minutes before manipulation and disinfect it three times with concentrated liquid soap and 70% alcohol soaked in gauze. Protect the workbench with sterile material that does not release particles;
- Keep inside the cabin a specific rigid container (descartex II) for the disposal of contaminated material.
- Wash your hands aseptically and dress yourself before any procedure.

- Disinfect the ampoule necks, the rubber caps of the vials, and the infusion solution injector with a sterile swab and antiseptic solution, using repeated unidirectional movements;
- Protect the insertion site of the needle into the vial with a sterile swab in order to avoid possible release of splashes or aerosols onto the workbench;
- Vial

-Freeze-dried:

-After the rubber stopper of the vial and the ampoule of diluent have been aseptically capped, aspirate the necessary volume of diluent for reconstitution of the lyophilized product.

-Pierce the rubber stopper of the vial (position the needle at 45°) and introduce the syringe volume slowly down the wall of the vial to avoid aerosolization and foaming.

-Remove any remaining solution from the syringe and needle (position the needle inside the vial in a solution-free space and aspirate a portion of air) and disconnect the needle from the vial using a sterile compress as protection.

-Reconstitute the drug, with or without agitation (as directed by the manufacturer), and aspirate the necessary volume, according to the prescribed dose, respecting the internal pressure of the vial (introduce air if necessary).

-If the cytotoxic is dispensed into the syringe, cap it with a luer lock device after discarding the needle. This device prevents accidents during transportation of the medication.

-If the drug needs to be diluted in another solution, disinfect the needle insertion site. Be careful not to puncture the diluent bag.Connect the line to the inside of the cabin and, as a safety measure, fill only with diluent solution before introducing the drug.If the volume of diluent is greater than prescribed, discard it in an appropriate container (beaker) inside the cabin, taking precautions against possible contamination.After introducing the drug, disinfect the puncture site again with sterile gauze and alcohol 70%.

-solution:

-disinfect the rubber cap, insert the needle, and aspirate the desired volume.

-Disconnect the needle from the vial and proceed in the same way as for the lyophilized medication already discontinued.

-Ampola:

-Disinfect the neck of the vial and remove possible volume of the solution present in the upper portion of the vial.

-Open the ampoule with compress protection in its neck to avoid accidents and possible aerosol formation.

-insert the bevel of the needle near the opening of the vial, facing the wall of the vial (avoid aspiration of shards).

-take out the required volume and return the excess to the vial to prevent bubbles from forming.

-transfer the contents of the syringe into a diluent solution as described above or,cap it with a luer lock device if the cytotoxic is dispensed into the syringe.

-Oral solids (tablets, capsules and lozenges):

-Manipulate inside the CBS wearing gloves, apron and mask.

-Avoid fragmentation and release of powders.

-Protect the manipulation site with a field.

-Do not use automatic counting machines to avoid contamination of the equipment and the work area.

-After manipulation, clean the area with soap and water followed by 70% alcohol.

-If it is necessary to crush the pills, place them in a sealed plastic bag and then crush them with a spoon or pistil, avoiding the rupture of the plastic bag.

-Inspect bags, vials or syringes with medication.Consider the presence of precipitates, leaks, color changes, total volume, proper identification and packaging.Seal the package to avoid any contamination from spillage during the transport process.

-Dispose of all contaminated material, including gloves, into the rigid container located inside the cabin. Seal and identify the container. Segregate in a specific area until it is collected and incinerated.

-Turn off the CBS at the end of all manipulations for the day at least 30 minutes after the last medication prepared.

Verification of refrigerator temperature and room temperature: Ensure the physical-chemical characteristics of the drugs as recommended by the manufacturer; detect temperature variations inside the refrigerator.

- Check the temperature every day, between 07:00 and 19:00.
- Always check the current temperature on the thermometer display. The letter out located in the upper corner of the lower display indicates that it refers to the refrigerator's temperature. The "in" sign found in the upper corner of the display indicates that it refers to the room temperature. Record the value on the Daily Temperature Recording Form in the corresponding field.
- To check the maximum and minimum temperatures, press the Max/Min button that will initially indicate the maximum temperature (the acronym Max should appear in the upper corner of the display) and press once more to show the minimum temperature (the acronym min should appear in the upper corner of the display). Record the value on the Daily Temperature Recording Form, in the respective fields.
- At the end of the logging press the reset button to update the Max/min values.
- Justify in the ``Additional remarks" field the temperatures that are outside the reference range (2 to 8°c) in the case of the refrigerator reading.
- Sign in the "Signature" field.

Paramentation for preparing drugs at the chemotherapy center: To guarantee the handler's safety; to guarantee the sterility of the manipulated product.

- Wash your hands using aseptic technique;
- Change your personal clothing to the hospital's standardized clothing;
- Put on the cap and put on the pro - feet;
- Bridging the physical barrier between the "dirty" area and the clean area;
- Perform hand and nail brushing using aseptic technique in the hygiene room;
- Put on a pair of procedure gloves;
- Put on the 3M 8801 respirator;
- Enter the antechamber;
- Put on the apron;
- Enter the handling room;

- Put on two pairs of sterile gloves, one pair on top of the other, before handling the cytostatics.

Control of drugs controlled by Ordinance 344 in the oncology/SUS ambulatory: Control the dispensing of drugs regulated by Ordinance 344 of May 12, 1998; register the preparations of controlled drugs in the dilution center; keep stock control up to date.

- Receive the prescription for controlled medication from the nursing staff;
- Make the label according to SOP DFINQUIM004;
- Inform and ask the pharmacist to remove the medication from the cabinet of controlled drugs, according to Ordinance 344;
- Take the label and medication to the manipulation room for preparation (in the case of injectables) and subsequent dispensing to the nursing staff.
- File the 2nd copy of the prescription in a specific folder (for manual prescriptions);
- Record in the Specific Record book: date of preparation or administration, complete name of the patient, prescribed dose, person responsible for the preparation or record, signature and stamp. And when it is an electronic prescription, write down its number.

Contingency plan for the chemotherapy refrigerator: Establish rules to be followed in case of temperature deviations, due to technical problems with equipment and/or power outages; ensure safe storage of thermolabile drugs.

-Power outage

- Check and note the refrigerator's temperature right after the power failure;
- Avoid opening the refrigerator;
- Constantly monitor the temperature (15 minute interval0 and note the fluctuations on the log sheet on the observation board;
- If the temperature is outside the specified range (2 to 8°c), transfer the drugs to a thermos box previously packed with icex and monitor the temperature;
- In case of temperature loss to the environment (temperature rise), add a few more units of icex in the cooler box;

- Forward the medications for temporary storage in a fully functioning refrigerator;
- Contact maintenance.

- Temperature deviation outside the ideal range

- If the temperature deviates from the ideal range (2 to 8/c), the refrigerator's power must be adjusted as needed. The thermostat is located on the outside of the refrigerator;
- Wait a few minutes for the internal temperature of the equipment to stabilize;
- If the temperature does not stabilize, transfer the drugs to a thermos box previously packed with icex and forward to a refrigerator that is in full operation, and communicate maintenance for necessary adjustments of the refrigerator;
- Record the temperature deviation in the observation frame of the Temperature Recording Sheet.

PROTOCOL TYPES

All protocols have preparations with serotherapy, salts, corticoids and antiemetics, some with antihistamines.

- CMF: CTX (D1) + MTX (D1) + 5FU (D1)
- AC: ADM (D1) + CTX (D1)
- TOPOTECAN (D1-D5)
- PACLITAXEL WEEKLY (D1-D8-D15)
- VINORELBINE (D1-D8-D15)
- FAC: 5FU (D1)+ADM (D1)+CTX (D1)
- 5FU+LV (MAYO CLINI) (D1-D5)
- GENCITABINE (D1-D8-D15) 1000 MG/M^2
- CARBOPLATIN (D1)+PACLITAXEL (D1)
- CISPLATIN (D1)+PACLITAXEL (D1)
- ELF: VP(D1-D3)+5FU (D1-D3)+LV (D1-D3)
- CISPLATIN (D1)+ETOPOSITE (D1-D3)
- MITOXANTRONE (D1)
- DOCETAXEL (D1) 75 MG/M^2
- CDDP (D1)+GEMZAR (D1-D8)- BILIARY V.
- PEB: VP (D1-D5)+CDDP (D1-D5)+BLEO (D2-D9-D16)
- CDDP (D1)+ADM (D1-D2-D3)- OSTEOSARCOMA
- WEEKLY CDDP (D1-D8-D15) 40 MG/M^2 - UTERINE C.
- CDDP (D1) FULL DOSE
- TC: DOCETAXEL (D1)+CTX (D1)
- FLOX-OXA: OXA (D1) + 5FU (D1-D2) + LV (D1-D2)
- FLOX - OXA/ 5FU/LV:
- 5FU+LV (WEEKLY) ROSWELL PARK
- IC: CPTII (D1-D8)+CDDP (D1-D8)
- MTX WEEKLY
- IFL: CPTII + 5FU (D1-D8-D15-D22)
- COP: CTX + VCR (D1)+ PDN (D1-D5) (HEMATO)

101

- ABVD: ADM+BLEO+VLB+DTIC (D1-D15) (HEMATO)
- COP: CTX+ADM+VCR (D1)+PDN (D1-D5) (HEMATO)
- R-CHOP; RITUXIMAB+CTX+ADM+VCR (D1) (HEMATO)
- DOCETAXEL (D1-D8-D15) 30 MG/M^2
- CDDP (D1-D8) + GEMZAR (D1-D8)BREAST
- CDDP (D1)+ADM (D1) ENDOMETRIUM
- CDDP (D1-D8)+ VP (D1 TO D5) (C/RT)
- CDDP (D1)+PACLITAXEL (D1-D8-D15)
- CARBOPLATIN (D1)+PACLITAXEL (D1-D8-D15)
- TAMOXYFEN
- FASLODEX
- ANASTROZOLE
- BICALUTAMIDE
- CYPROTERONE
- LUPRON 3.75 MG
- XELOA
- MTX+VLB (D1-D8-D15-D22)
- DTIC (1000 MG/M^2 D1)
- CDDP WEEKLY 30 MG/M^2 (D1-D8-D15)
- WEEKLY FLOX
- IFOSFAMIDE (D1 TO D5)+ADM (D1 TO D3)
- FILGRASTIM 300 MCG (D1 TO D5)
- PAMIDRONATE 90 MG
- PAMIDRONATE 90 MG
- PACLITAXEL WEEKLY (D1-D8-D15-D22)
- WEEKLY MTX (D1-D8-D15) 180 MG/M^2 - INVASIVE SPRING
- FILGRASTIM 300 MCG (D2 TO D8)
- VAC: VCR+CTX+ADM+MESNA (D1)
- DTIC 250 MG/M^2 (D1 TO D5)
- GEMCITABINE (D1-D8)+PACLITAXEL (D1)
- WEEKLY ADM
- PCV: LOMUSTINE+PROCARBAZINE+VCR

- PACLITAXEL +CARBOPLATIN (D1-D8) - CA ESOPHAGUS
- LUPRON 7.5 MG
- GENCITABINE (D1-D8)+DOCETAXEL (D8) - SARCOMAS
- HERCEPTIN 1ST INFUSION
- HERCEPTIN 2ND AND SUBSEQUENT DOSES
- ONCO BCG

PALLIATIVE CARE

Palliative Care, according to the National Academy of Palliative Care (ANCP) is undoubtedly the exercise of the art of caring allied to scientific knowledge, in which the association of science and art provides the relief of suffering related to the disease. As a fundamental part of clinical practice, it may occur in parallel to therapies aimed at the cure and prolongation of life.

Palliative Care, due to the complex, multidimensional, and dynamic nature of the disease, advances as a therapeutic model that addresses the look and therapeutic proposal to the diverse symptoms responsible for the physical, psychological, spiritual, and social suffering, responsible for diminishing the quality of life of the patient. It is a growing area whose progress comprises diverse strategies that encompass bioethics, communication, and the nature of suffering.

The age range is independent of the need for this care, since it is a universal type of care, which is extended to the patient and his family. Palliative Care must focus on the adequate evaluation and handling of the physical, psychological, social, and spiritual symptoms of the patient and his family, and be present in all phases of the disease trajectory. There is a greater understanding of disease and symptom mechanisms and the various therapeutic options for physical and psychological symptoms (National Academy of Palliative Care (ANCP).

REFERENCES

NATIONAL ACADEMY OF PALLIATIVE CARE (ANCP). Manual de cuidados paliativos. Rio de Janeiro: Diagraphic, 2009.

ALMEIDA, José Ricardo Chamhum de. PHARMACISTS IN ONCOLOGY. Atheneu: 2010. 2nd Edition.

ANVISA (Agência Nacional de Vigilância Sanitária). [online] Banco de Dados de Medicamentos. Available at: http://www.anvisa.gov.br/medicamentos/base. Access: 11 May 2023.

ANVISA (National Health Surveillance Agency). [online] Bulário Eletrônico. Available at: http://www.anvisa.gov.br/fila_bula/. Accessed on 11 May 2023.

ALMEIDA, José Ricardo Chamhun. Pharmacists in Oncology: a new reality / 2nd edition - São Paulo: Editora Atheneu, 2010.

Pharmaceutical Laboratories' Package Leaflets in Oncology.

Drug Information Handbook; 15th Edition; Page 726.

ATHAUFO DE PAIVA FOUNDATION (FAP). Imuno BCG complete package insert. Available at: http://www.bcgfap.com.br/web/bula-completa-imuno-bcg/. Accessed on 11 May 2023.

Guia Farmacêutico 2012-2013, Hospital Sírio Libanês - 6th edition printed in January/2012.

Dilution Guide, Eurofarma Laboratory.

NATIONAL INSTITUTE OF CANCER (INCA) What is cancer. Available at: www2. inca.gov.br/wps/wcm/connect/cancer/site/oquee. Accessed May 11, 2023.

ONCOGUIA INSTITUTE. Learn how to face the side effects. Available at:

http://www.oncoguia.org.br/conteudo/nauseas-e-vomitos/1334/109/. Accessed May 11, 2023.

Oncology Line Reference Material, Libbs Laboratory - April 2012 Edition.

TRISSEL, L.A. Handbook on injectable drugs. 16. ed. Bethesda, Maryland: American Society of Health-System Pharmacists, 2011. BUZAID, A.C.; MALUF, F.C.; LIMA, C.M.R.

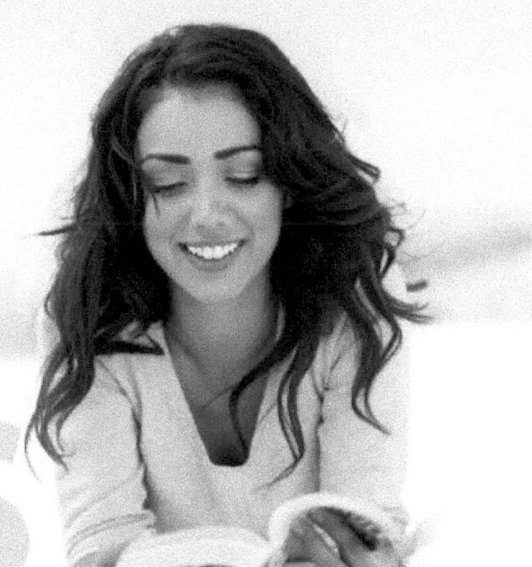

Buy your books fast and straightforward online - at one of world's fastest growing online book stores! Environmentally sound due to Print-on-Demand technologies.

Buy your books online at
www.morebooks.shop

Kaufen Sie Ihre Bücher schnell und unkompliziert online – auf einer der am schnellsten wachsenden Buchhandelsplattformen weltweit! Dank Print-On-Demand umwelt- und ressourcenschonend produziert.

Bücher schneller online kaufen
www.morebooks.shop

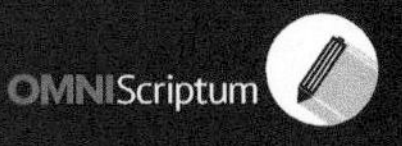

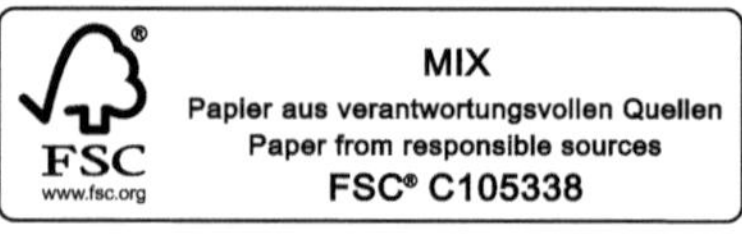